Video Atlas of Laparoscopic Surgery

Bariatric Surgery

System requirements:

- **Operating System—Windows Vista or above**
- **Web Browser—Google Chrome, Mozilla Firefox, Internet Explorer 9 and above**
- **Essential plugins—Java & Flash Player**
  - If you are experiencing problems viewing content, please check that your system has Java enabled.
  - If the video clips do not appear, your system may require Flash Player or require an update to Flash Player settings. To learn more about Flash Player settings, please click on the link in the "Help" section of the CD/DVD.
  - You can test Java and Flash Player by using the associated links available in the "Help" section of the CD/DVD.

Please note that this CD/DVD will only play in a computer or laptop and will not work properly in a DVD player.

This CD/DVD come with an "Autorun" function; it may take a few seconds to load on your computer. If the content does not load, please follow the steps listed below to access the contents manually:

- Click on "My Computer".
- Select the CD/DVD drive and Click "Open/Explore". A list of available files will appear.
- Find and double click the file "launch.html".

For more information about troubleshooting, please click on http://support.microsoft.com/kb/330135.

Video Atlas of Laparoscopic Surgery

Bariatric Surgery

Vol. 1

Editor

Rana C Pullatt MD MS MRCS FACS
Director Bariatric Surgery VISN-7
Associate Profesor of Surgery
Director Robotic Surgery
Medical University of South Carolina
Charleston, South Carolina, USA

Foreword

Robin P Blackstone MD FACS

JAYPEE *The Health Sciences Publisher*

New Delhi | London | Philadelphia | Panama

Jaypee Brothers Medical Publishers (P) Ltd

Headquarters
Jaypee Brothers Medical Publishers (P) Ltd.
4838/24, Ansari Road, Daryaganj
New Delhi 110 002, India
Phone: +91-11-43574357
Fax: +91-11-43574314
E-mail: jaypee@jaypeebrothers.com

Overseas Offices

J.P. Medical Ltd.
83, Victoria Street, London
SW1H 0HW (UK)
Phone: +44-20 3170 8910
Fax: +44(0)20 3008 6180
E-mail: info@jpmedpub.com

Jaypee Medical Inc.
The Bourse
111 South Independence Mall East
Suite 835
Philadelphia, PA 19106, USA
Phone: +1 267-519-9789
E-mail: jpmed.us@gmail.com

Jaypee Brothers Medical Publishers (P) Ltd.
Bhotahity, Kathmandu, Nepal
Phone: +977-9741283608
E-mail: kathmandu@jaypeebrothers.com

Jaypee-Highlights Medical Publishers Inc.
City of Knowledge, Bld. 237, Clayton
Panama City, Panama
Phone: +1 507-301-0496
Fax: +1 507-301-0499
E-mail: cservice@jphmedical.com

Jaypee Brothers Medical Publishers (P) Ltd.
17/1-B, Babar Road, Block-B, Shaymali
Mohammadpur, Dhaka-1207
Bangladesh
Mobile: +08801912003485
E-mail: jaypeedhaka@gmail.com

Website: www.jaypeebrothers.com
Website: www.jaypeedigital.com

Inquiries for bulk sales may be solicited at: jaypee@jaypeebrothers.com

Video Atlas of Laparoscopic Surgery—Bariatric Surgery (Vol. 1)

First Edition: **2016**

ISBN: 978-93-5152-935-4

Printed at: Ajanta Offset & Packagings Ltd., New Delhi

Dedication

To my best friend and wife Arasi and our precious kids Arjun, Yuvan and Raeya from whom I have spent countless hours away practicing my craft. Surgery is indeed a jealous mistress.

To my parents, Raman and Lakshmi and my brother, Raj. I have the deepest gratitude for always being there for me.

Contributors

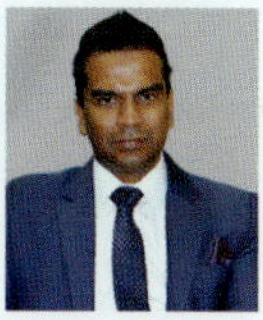

Rana C Pullatt MD MS MRCS FACS is an Associate Professor of Surgery at the Medical University of South Carolina. He serves as the Director of Robotic Surgery and is the Associate Director for Surgical Simulation at the Medical University of South Carolina, USA. He also serves as the Director of Bariatric Surgery for VISN-7. He has made several National and International presentations in Bariatrics and Advanced Laparoendoscopic Surgery. He is the lead author and editor for this Video Atlas.

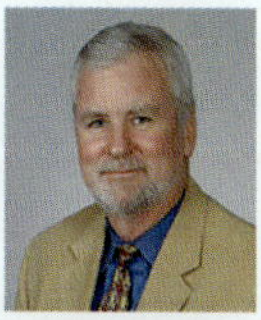

T Karl Byrne MD FACS is a Professor of Surgery and is one of the most experienced Bariatric Surgeons in South Carolina. He serves as the Medical Director of Bariatric Surgery at the Medical University of South Carolina, USA.

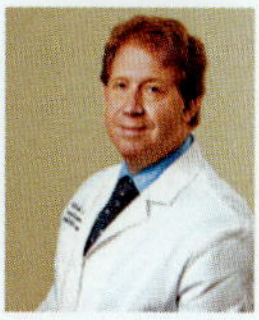

Mitch Roslin MD FACS serves as the Director of Bariatric Surgery at Lenox Hill Hospital and at the Northern Westchester Hospital System New York, USA. He has authored several publications and is considered a world renowned expert in the Laparoscopic Duodenal Switch and the SIPS procedure.

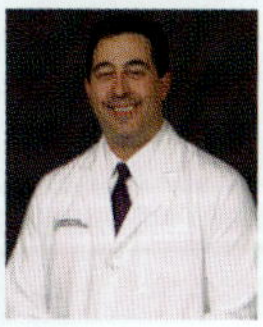

John Scott MD FACS FASMBS is a clinical Associate Professor of Surgery at the University of South Carolina, USA. He serves as the Fellowship Program Director and is the Program Director for Bariatric Surgery at the Greenville Hospital System, South Carolina, USA.

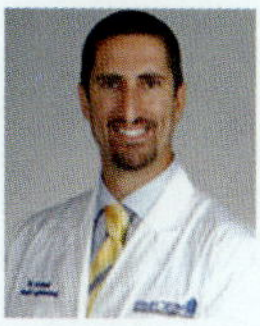

Greg Cote MD FACS is an Associate Professor of Medicine in the Division of Gastroenterology at the Medical University of South Carolina, USA. He has authored several publications and is an expert in ERCP and Interventional endoscopy.

Foreword

It gives me great pleasure to write a foreword for the *Video Atlas of Laparoscopic Surgery—Bariatric Surgery* edited by surgeon, Rana C Pullatt, MD MS MRCS FACS.

The twin epidemics of obesity and type 2 diabetes are increasing, type 2 diabetes mellitus affects over 366 million people in the world (8.3%). In China, type 2 diabetes and prediabetes have a prevalence of 11.6% and 50.1% respectively affecting 113.9 million and 493.4 million people. Metabolic and Bariatric Surgery (MBS) plays an important role in preserving life and health of individuals affected by obesity and type 2 diabetes and is an important vehicle for tertiary prevention including progression of prediabetes to diabetes, cardiovascular disease and cancer.

Although participating in fellowship training is ideal, with so many people affected many surgeons will need to learn these techniques in a setting of postgraduate education that does not include fellowship. In this situation, safety becomes a primary concern.

The American Society for Metabolic and Bariatric Surgery (ASMBS), the Society of American Gastrointestinal and Endoscopic Surgeons and the International Federation for the Surgery of Obesity and Metabolic Disorders offer peer reviewed on line videos of MBS techniques that require Internet access. There is a need therefore for a comprehensive video atlas in a technically challenging field like MBS that can be accessed from anywhere in the world, even where there is little or no Internet access. This atlas fills that niche well. The videos are well edited, highlighting the technical nuances of performing MBS procedures and offering a variety of techniques and approaches to mitigate training bias.

In addition to technical excellence, surgeons, who provide surgical care for the patient with obesity, must establish a multidisciplinary approach that adhere to the principles established by the Metabolic and Bariatric Surgery Assessment and Quality Improvement Program, including tracking outcomes in all patients. Surgeons should augment the Video Atlas technical instruction with study data on the risks, benefits and long-term consequences of MBS to enable them to achieve adequate informed consent for surgery. Surgeons should also attend high quality organized educational meetings available through local surgical societies in most parts of the world.

My hope is that use of this volume along with the next volume of this atlas, incorporating Revisional Bariatric Surgery, will prove to enhance the surgeon's education by offering a comprehensive resource of techniques in this field. I encourage surgeons and fellows who wish to incorporate metabolic and bariatric surgery in their practice do so in a safe and effective manner in the context of a strong program of care.

Robin P Blackstone MD FACS
Associate Clinical Professor of Surgery
University of Arizona School of Medicine-Phoenix
Past President, American Society for
Metabolic and Bariatric Surgery
Banner University Medical Center, Phoenix, Arizona, USA

Preface

This Atlas is a result of my own quest in performing safe bariatric surgery. My technique over the years of performing these operations has evolved and I have learnt immensely from watching several master surgeons at other institutes. During my training, I learnt the retrocolic retrogastric approach of doing a laparoscopic gastric bypass. Although I am convinced in its use in the super morbidly obese, I believe as bariatric surgeons we must be familiar in different ways of doing the same operation. All mainstream bariatric operations are detailed in this Atlas with narratives, port positions, and pictures along with edited videos, which highlight technical details and nuances in performing these complex operations. I am hopeful this Atlas will help a surgeon who is in practice, perfect his technique and also familiarize him/her with another way of doing the same operation if the need arises. I also believe this Atlas will be extremely useful for Residents and Fellows in-training to absorb the technical details of these operations in a more relaxed pace at their own time. I hope this Atlas will supplement and help with the steep learning curve of traditional training in Bariatric Surgery.

Rana C Pullatt MD MS MRCS FACS
Director Bariatric Surgery VISN-7
Associate Profesor of Surgery
Director Robotic Surgery
Medical University of South Carolina
Charleston, South Carolina, USA

Acknowledgments

I would like to thank Professor Prabhakar Baliga for training me and molding me into the surgeon I am today.

I would like to thank Professor David Adams for his mentorship and support.

I would like to acknowledge the contributions of my esteemed co-authors Mitch Roslin, T Karl Byrne and John Scott for their invaluable contributions to the making of this atlas.

I would like to thank JS Rajkumar for sparking my interest in Minimally Invasive Surgery and starting me on this journey.

I would like to thank Chetna Malhotra Vohra (Associate Director) for conceptualizing and getting this project into fruition.

This Atlas would have been impossible but for the tireless work by Sheetal Arora Kapoor (Development Editor) and I am indebted to her.

Lastly, I would also like to thank Mr Jitendar P Vij (Group Chairman), Mr Ankit Vij (Group President) and Production team of Jaypee Brothers Medical Publishers (P) Ltd., New Delhi, India.

Contents

Video Content List

Chapter 1: Laparoscopic Sleeve Gastrectomy—This video describes in technical detail salient points in performing an ideal sleeve gastrectomy. —Rana C Pullatt MD MS MRCS FACS

Chapter 2: Laparoscopic Gastric Bypass—Circular Anastomosis using ORVIL—This video demonstrates salient technical details and tips in performing a gastric bypass using a transoral circular stapler. —Rana C Pullatt MD MS MRCS FACS

Chapter 3: Laparoscopic Antecolic Antegastric Bypass—This video demonstrates a simplified way in performing an antilock antegastirc Roux-en-Y gastric bypass.
—Rana C Pullatt MD MS MRCS FACS

Chapter 4: Laparoscopic Retrocolic Retrogastric Roux-en-Y Gastric Bypass—This video demonstrates tips in creating a mesocolic window and performing a gastric bypass in a super morbidly obese patient.
—Rana C Pullatt MD MS MRCS FACS, T Karl Byrne MD FACS

Chapter 5: Robotic Assisted Roux-en-Y Gastric Bypass—This video demonstrates performance of a single docking Roux-en-Y gastric bypass using the Davinci Si System.
—Rana C Pullatt MD MS MRCS FACS

Chapter 6: Laparoscopic Gastric Bypass—Circular Anastomosis Transgastric Method—This video demonstrates the introduction of a transgastric Anvil and performance of a circular anastomois.
—John Scott MD FACS FASMBS

Chapter 7: Laparoscopic Duodenal Switch—This video demonstrates the technical nuances and tips in performing a duodenal switch
—Mitch Roslin MD FACS

Chapter 8: ERCP in Roux-en-Y Gastric Bypass Patients—This video demonstrates the technical details of laparoscopic access of the excluded stomach and performance of an ERCP through this access port.
—Rana C Pullatt MD MS MRCS FACS, Greg Cote MD FACS

Chapter 9: SIPS (Stomach, Intestine and Pylorus Sparing Surgery)—This video demonstrates the technical details in performing a SIPS surgery. —Mitch Roslin MD FACS

1 Laparoscopic Sleeve Gastrectomy

Rana C Pullatt

OPERATIVE PROCEDURE

The patient is positioned supine with both arms out. An incision is made one open hand span width from the xiphoid process and two fingerbreadths to the left off the midline. This incision is deepened and the fascia is grasped with an Adair clamp. Pneumoperitoneum is introduced through a Veress needle to a pressure of 15 mm Hg. A 12 mm trocar is introduced through this. Diagnostic laparoscopy is performed. Alternatively in extremely obese patients a visual entry is done using a 12 mm trocar in the left subcostal region at palmers point using a visiport. A 5 mm trocar is placed just below the right costal margin in the anterior axillary line to introduce the liver retractor; alternatively the liver retractor can be placed just below the xiphoid process. A 5 mm trocar is placed on the right side just below the right costal margin at the midclavicular line. A 12 mm trocar is placed one hand width below that slightly to the right side of the 5 mm trocar. Two other trocars are placed in the left side. One 12 mm trocar is placed in the left subcostal margin in the midclavicular line. Another 5 mm trocar is placed one hand width below the 12 mm trocar. The angle of His is visualized and dissected (Fig. 1). The pylorus is identified. The greater curvature is marked 6 cm proximal to the pylorus. A spot in the greater curvature about midbody of the stomach is identified and the greater omentum is incised with an energy device and the lesser sac is entered (Figs. 2 and 3). The dissection of the greater omentum is continued cephalad to reach the short gastric vessels and the previously dissected angle of His (Fig. 4). The fundus is completely mobilized till the base of the left crus is visible. The greater omentum is then taken off the stomach in the caudal direction towards the mark placed 6 cm proximal to the pylorus. This completes the omental dissection. Once this is done a 38 French bougie is passed and is directed to the pylorus. Using the bougie as a guide stapling of the stomach is begun hugging the bougie and exerting even traction on the body of the stomach. Care is taken not to narrow the incisura too much (Fig. 5).

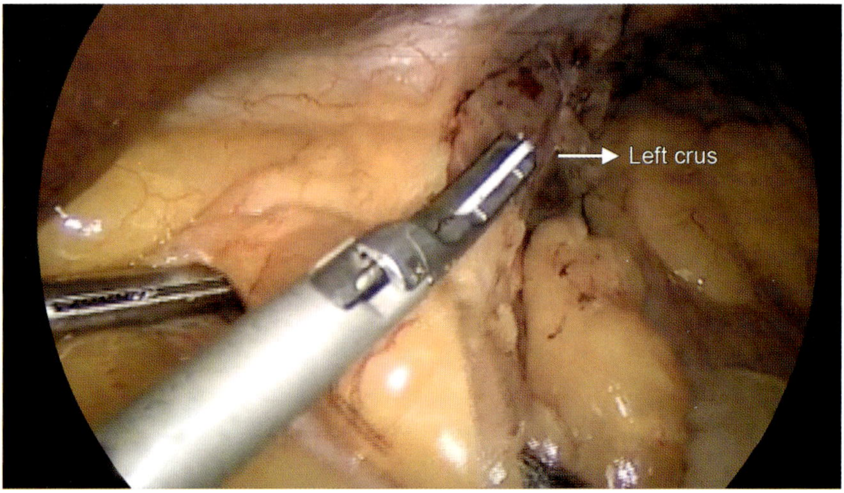

Fig. 1: Angle of His dissection.

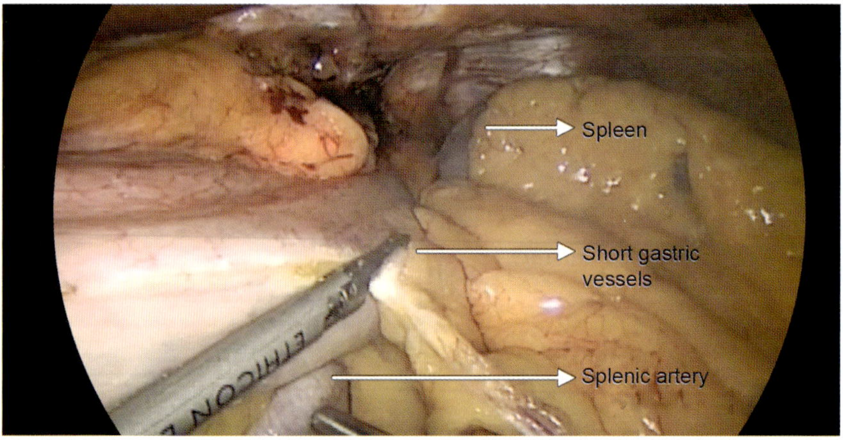

Fig. 2: Greater curvature dissection.

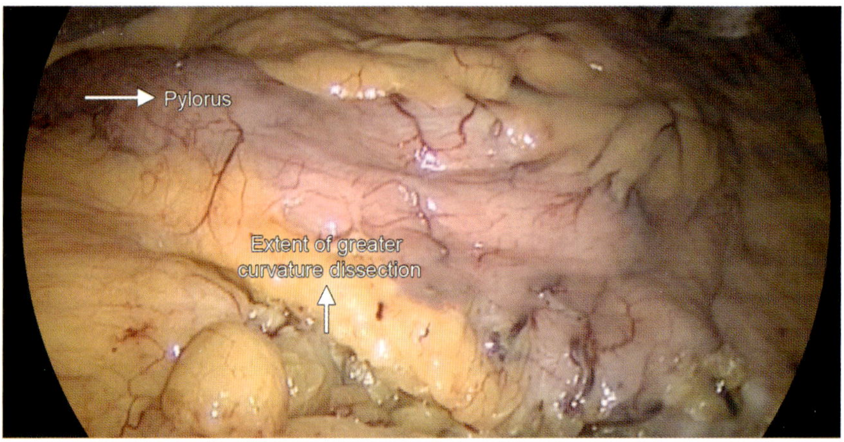

Fig. 3: Extent of greater curvature dissection.

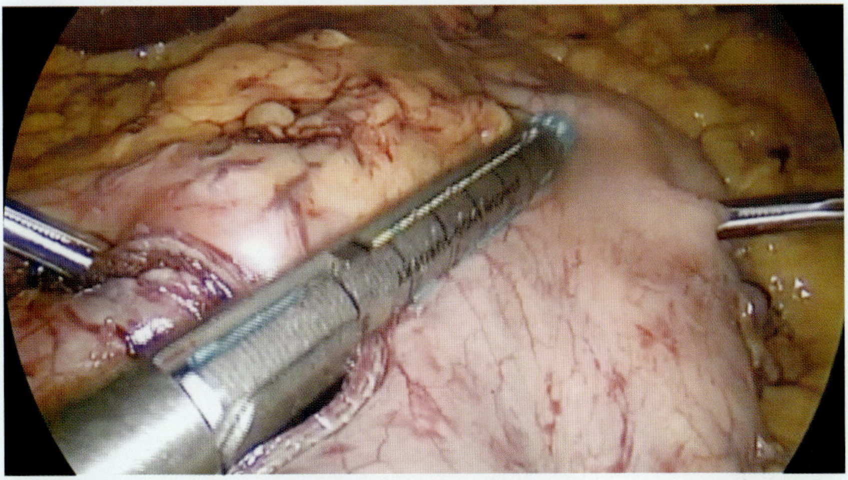

Fig. 4: Gastric division.

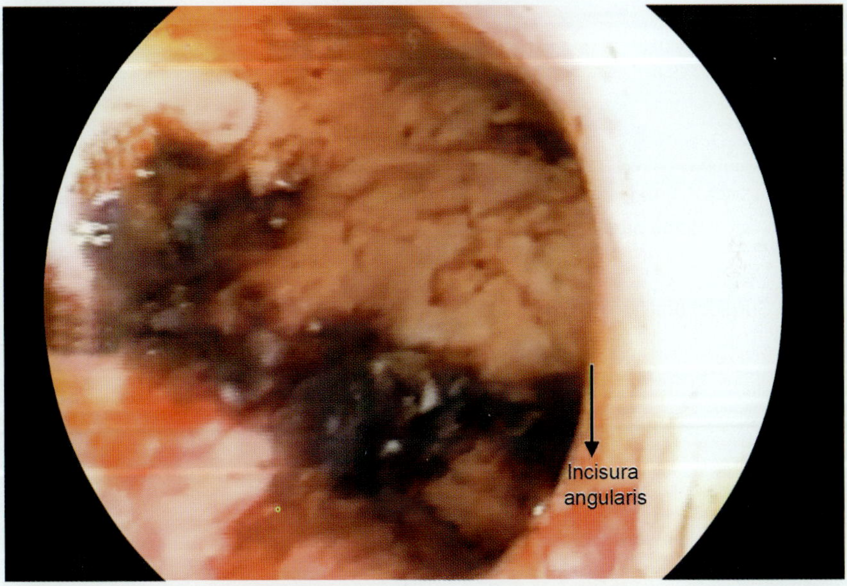

Fig. 5: Intraoperative endoscopy.

At all times anterior and posterior visualization of the stomach is done before stapling to ensure correct application of the stapler and to prevent spiraling of the sleeve. In the antral region nothing less than a thick tissue load is used to accomplish the division of the stomach. It is our practice to use a thick tissue load all the way up to the fundus. Alternatively a load one step below may be used for the fundus and the body of the stomach. Endoscopy is performed at the end of the operation to ensure that the sleeve is not narrowed and to ensure hemostasis. Patient positioning and trocar position is illustrated in Figures 6 and 7.

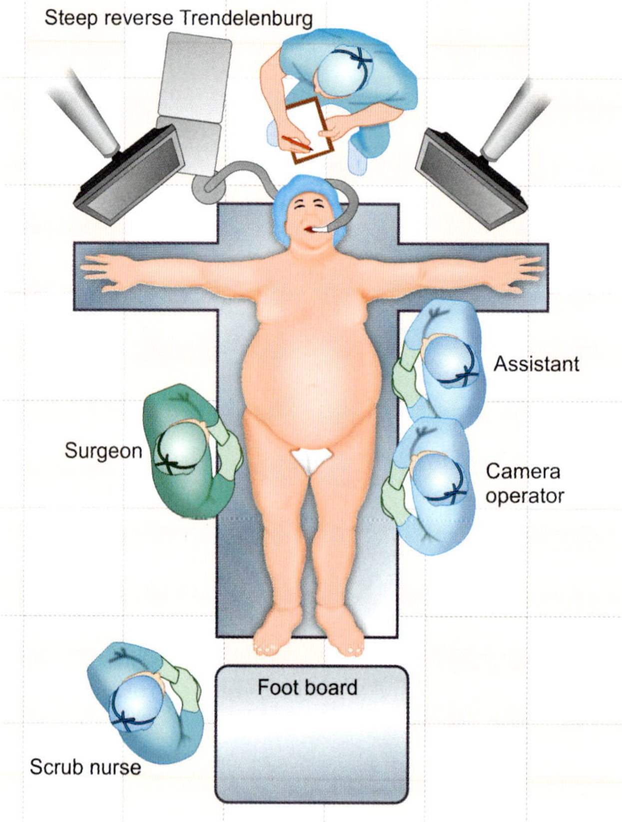

Fig. 6: Surgical positioning of patient.

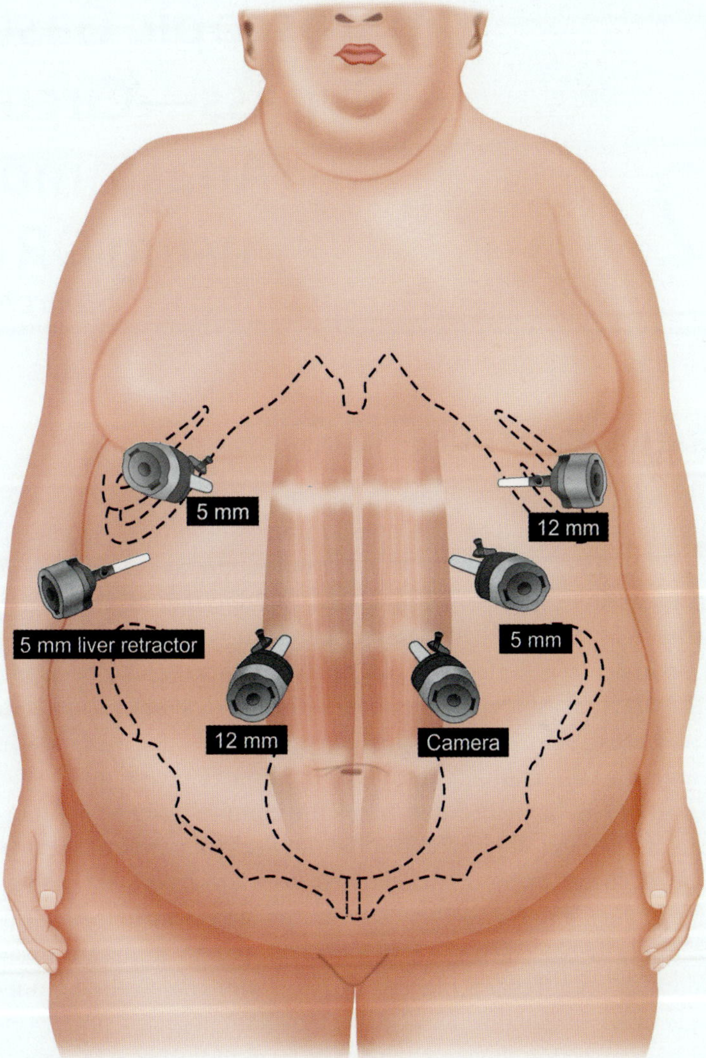

Fig. 7: Trocar position.

2

Laparoscopic Gastric Bypass—Circular Anastomosis using ORVIL

Rana C Pullatt

OPERATIVE PROCEDURE

The patient is positioned supine with both arms out. An incision is made one open hand span width from the xiphoid process and two fingerbreadths to the left off the midline. This incision is deepened and the fascia is grasped with an Adair clamp. Pneumoperitoneum is introduced through a Veress needle to a pressure of 15 mm Hg. A 12 mm trocar is introduced through this. Diagnostic laparoscopy is performed. Alternatively in extremely obese patients a visual entry is done using a 12 mm trocar in the left subcostal region at Palmer's point using a visiport. A 5 mm trocar is placed just below the right costal margin in the anterior axillary line to introduce the liver retractor; alternatively the liver retractor can be placed just below the xiphoid process. A 5 mm trocar is placed on the right side just below the right costal margin at the mid clavicular line. A 12 mm trocar is placed one hand width below that slightly to the right side of the 5 mm trocar. Two other trocars are placed in the left side. One 12 mm trocar is placed in the left subcostal margin in the mid clavicular line. Another 5 mm trocar is placed one hand width below the 12 mm trocar. The angle of His is visualized and dissected. A small gastric pouch (Fig. 1) is created by transecting the stomach at the level of the second gastric vessel about 5 cm from the GE junction in a perigastric fashion. A small L shaped pouch is thus created based on the lesser curvature. The ligament of Treitz is identified and the bowel is followed for 50 cm. The bowel is divided with a white load stapler and the biliary limb is marked with a clip. The mesenteric division is then achieved with a harmonic scalpel. The greater omentum if substantial is divided in front of the transverse colon using the harmonic scalpel. The 25 ORVIL is passed by the anesthesiologist as described in the video (Fig. 2). The ET tube cuff may be deflated for easy passage of the ORVIL in the hypopharynx. A small gastrotomy is performed on the pouch to enable passage of the ORVIL through the gastrotomy. The Anvil when adequately positioned in the gastric pouch is detached from the delivery mechanism by dividing the sutures that hold the Anvil to the tube (Fig. 3). The delivery mechanism of the ORVIL is extracted through the left upper quadrant 12 mm port. The end of the Roux limb is opened by excising the staple line. The 12 mm left upper quadrant is then removed. The port site may be dilated using Hegar dilators. The shaft of the EEA stapler is then introduced through this port site and is threaded into the end of the Roux limb. The EEA stapler spike is then deployed to exit the antimesenteric side of the Roux limb. The stapler is then mated to the Anvil and thus deployed (Fig. 4). The end of the Roux limb is stapled flush with the gastrojejunostomy completing the anastomosis. The Roux limb is then rotated in an anticlockwise direction for 100 cm. This point is then used to reanastomose the Roux limb and the biliary limb. This is done in a side-to-side fashion after jejunotomies are performed and a side-to-side anastomosis is fashioned after a single fire of the linear stapler with a white load (Fig. 5). The common enterotomy is closed with another fire of the stapler with a blue load; (Fig. 6) alternatively the common enterotomy can be closed with a 2-0 Vicryl. The mesenteric defect is closed using a 2-0 silk suture (Fig. 7). An antiobstruction Brolin stitch is placed at the jejunojejunostomy (Fig. 8). Petersen's space is closed using a 2-0 silk suture (Fig. 9). The gastrojejunal anastomosis is checked with an endoscope for hemostasis and an air leak test, this completes the procedure. Patient positioning and trocar position is illustrated in Figures 10 and 11.

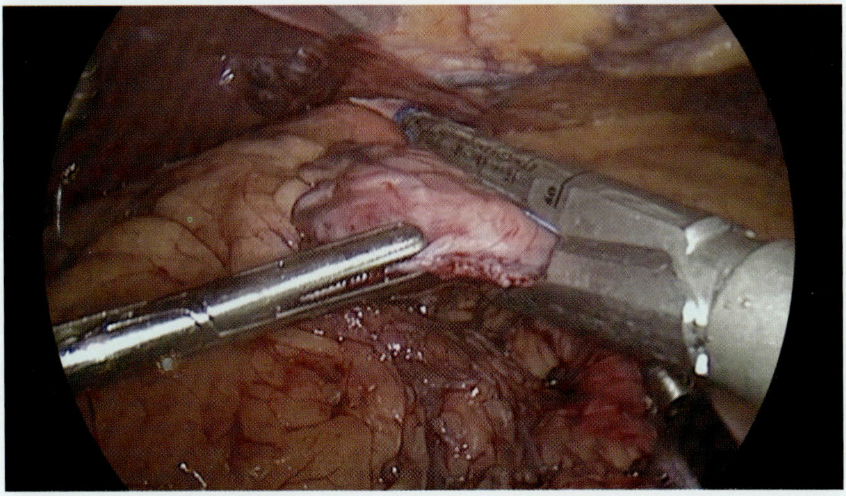

Fig. 1: Creation gastric pouch.

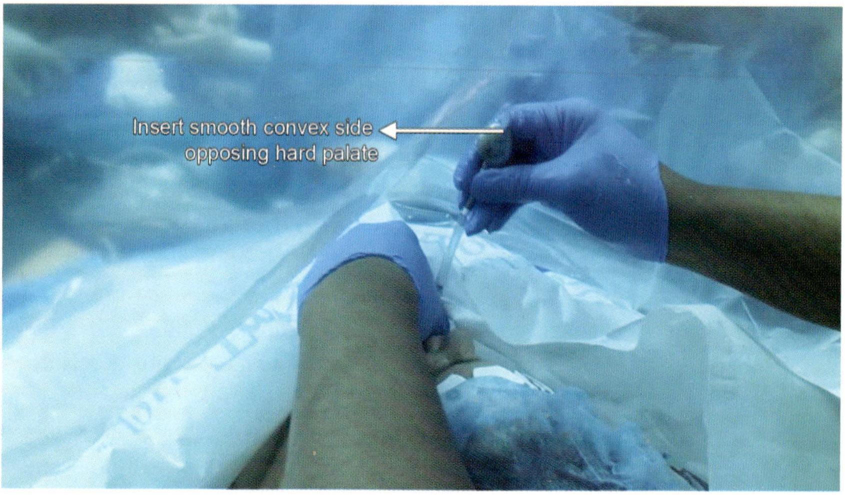

Fig. 2: ORVIL insertion.

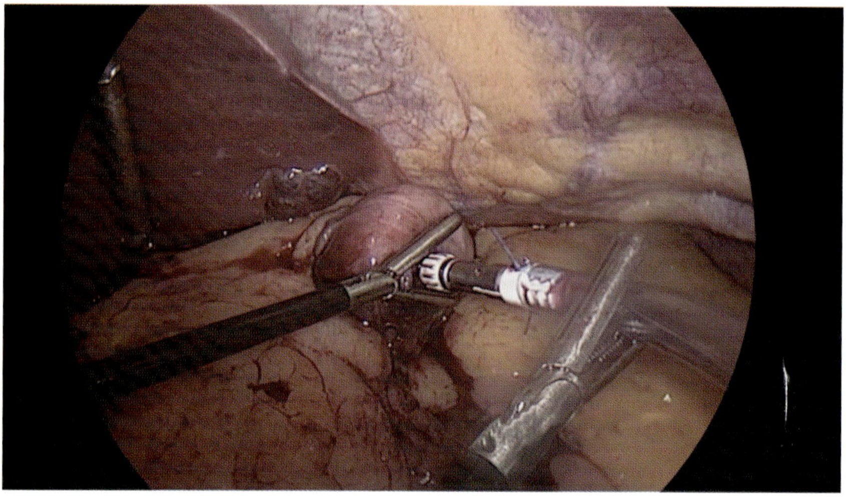

Fig. 3: Removal of ORVIL delivery mechanism.

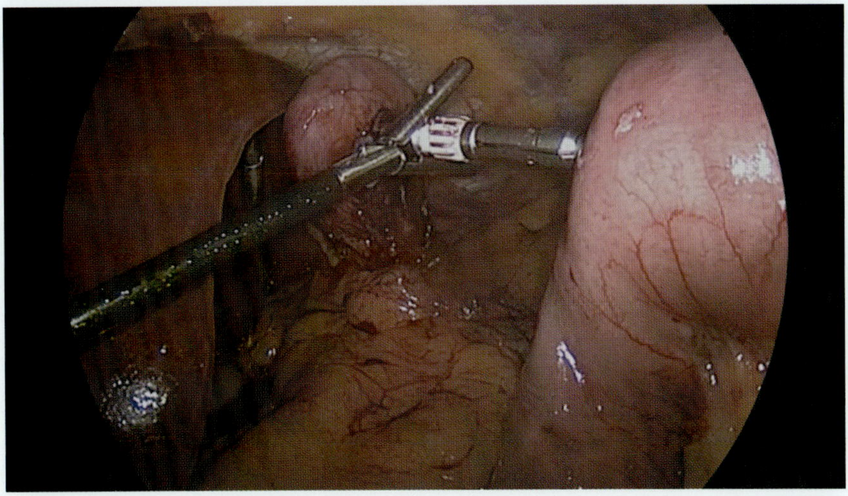

Fig. 4: Creation of gastrojejunostomy with 25 ORVIL DST.

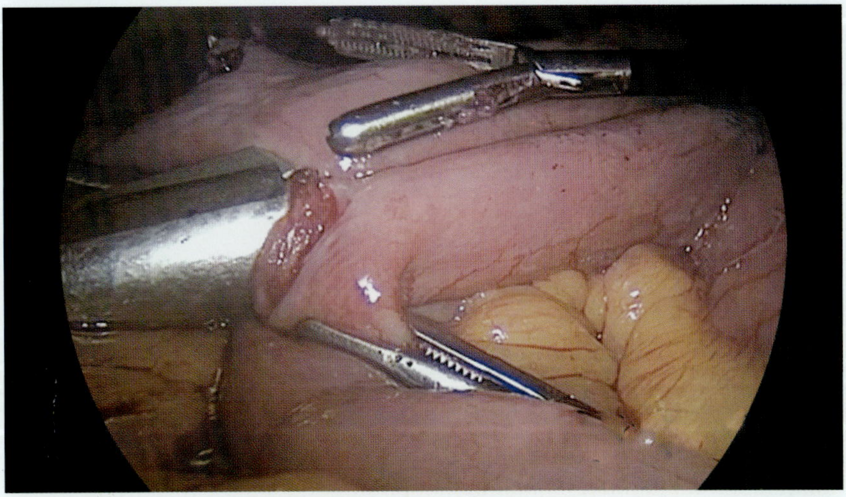

Fig. 5: Creation of jejunojejunostomy.

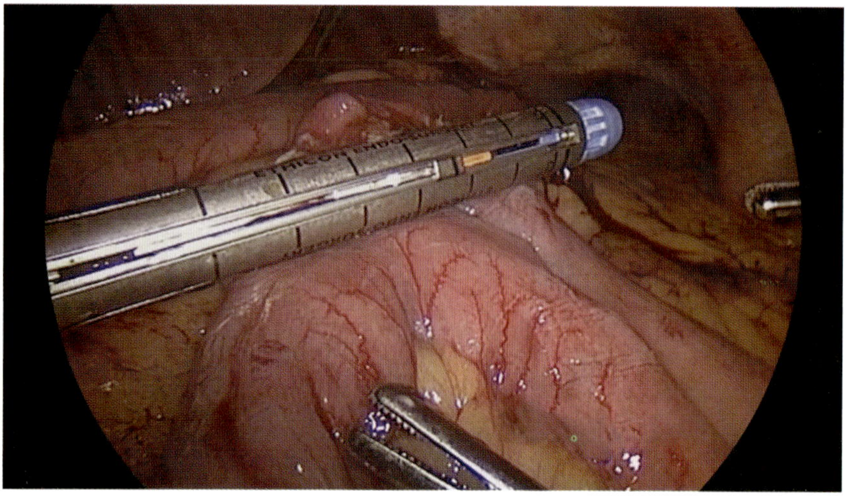

Fig. 6: Closure common enterotomy of jejunojejunostomy.

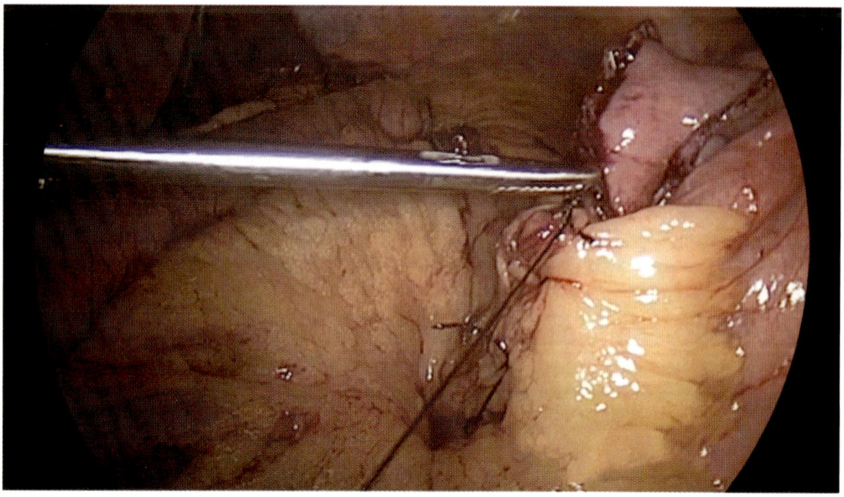

Fig. 7: Closure jejunojejunal mesenteric defect.

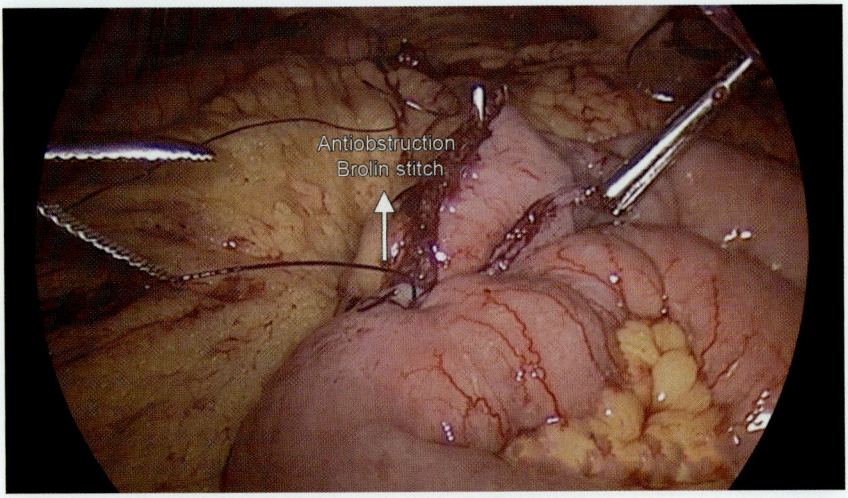

Fig. 8: Antiobstruction Brolin stitch.

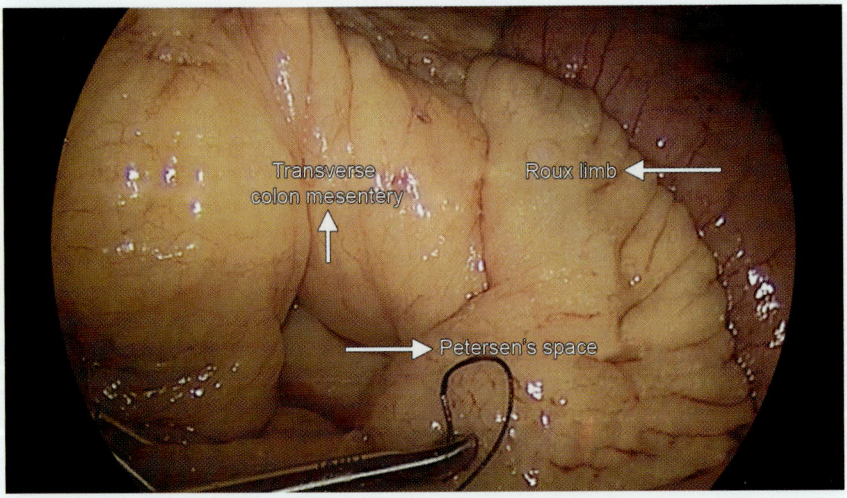

Fig. 9: Petersen's space closure.

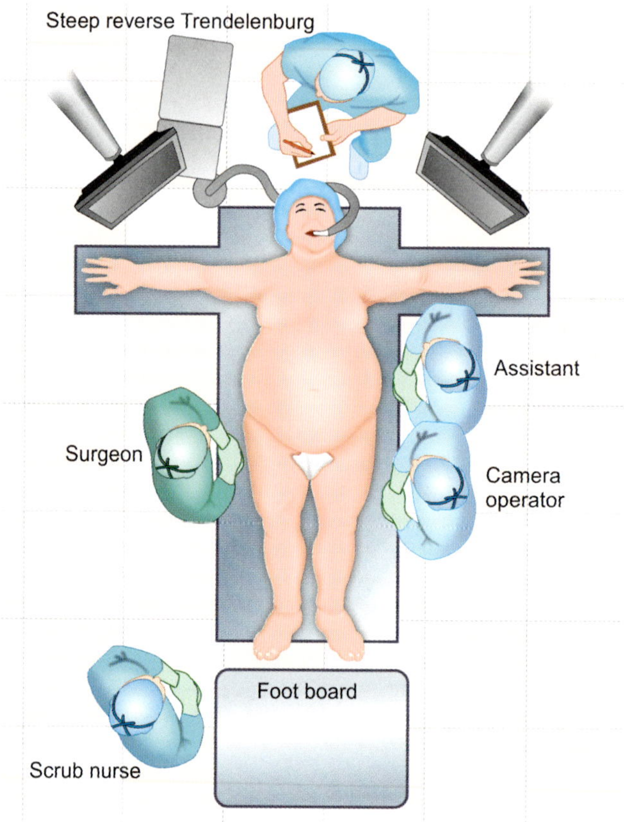

Fig. 10: Surgical positioning of patient.

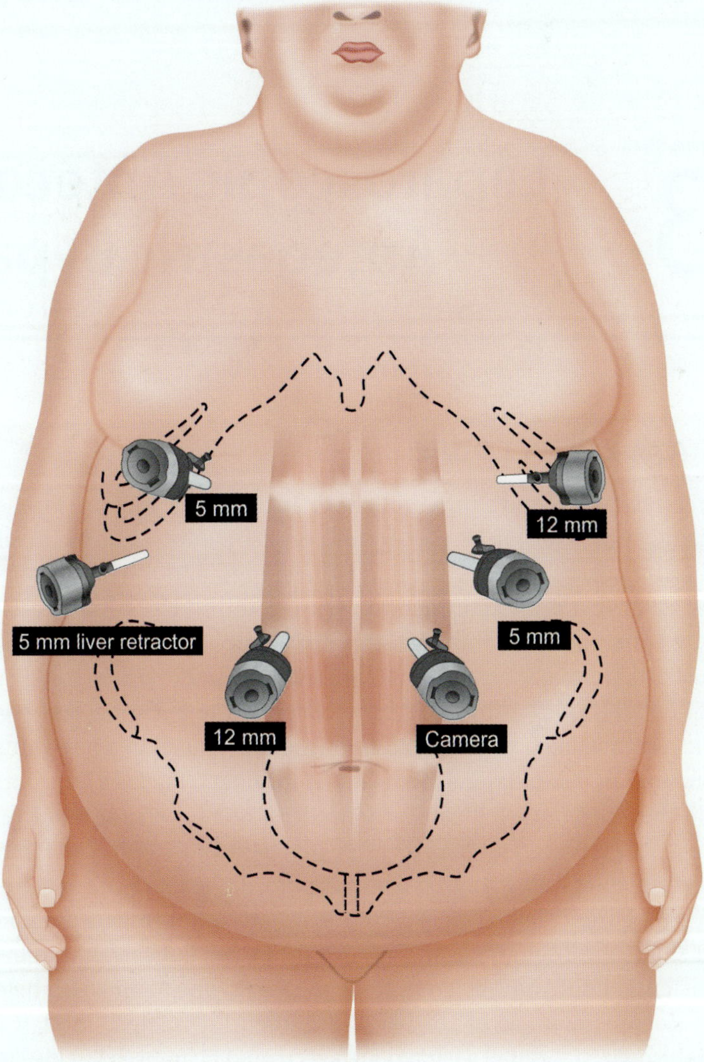

Fig. 11: Trocar position.

3 Laparoscopic Antecolic Antegastric Bypass

Rana C Pullatt

OPERATIVE PROCEDURE

The patient is positioned supine with both arms out. An incision is made one open hand span width from the xiphoid process and two fingerbreadths to the left off the midline. This incision is deepened and the fascia is grasped with an Adair clamp. Pneumoperitoneum is introduced through a Veress needle to a pressure of 15 mm Hg. A 12 mm trocar is introduced through this. Diagnostic laparoscopy is performed. Alternatively in extremely obese patients a visual entry is done using a 12 mm trocar in the left subcostal region at Palmer's point using a visiport. A 5 mm trocar is placed just below the right costal margin in the anterior axillary line to introduce the liver retractor; alternatively the liver retractor can be placed just below the xiphoid process. A 5 mm trocar is placed on the right side just below the right costal margin at the mid clavicular line. A 12 mm trocar is placed one hand width below that, slightly to the right side of the 5 mm trocar. Two other trocars are placed in the left side. One 12 mm trocar is placed in the left subcostal margin in the mid clavicular line. Another 5 mm trocar is placed one hand width below the 12 mm trocar. The angle of His is visualized and dissected. The left gastric artery is visualized. A small gastric pouch is created by transecting the stomach at the level of the second gastric vessel about 5 cm from the GE junction. The mesentery of the stomach is taken with the stapler. A green load is used for thick male stomachs and a blue load is usually used for female stomachs. The first fire of the stapler is done with staple line reinforcement. A small L shaped pouch is thus created based on the lesser curvature. Once complete division of the stomach is accomplished, the posterior side of the gastric pouch is cleared off the fat and mesentery for an appropriate area for anastomosis. The greater omentum is split if needed (Fig. 1). It is our observation that in most cases the splitting of the greater omentum is redundant and can be omitted, thereby not having the added expense of a harmonic scalpel. The ligament of Treitz is identified and the bowel is followed for 50 cm. A loop of bowel 50 cm distal to the ligament of Treitz is then brought up without tension to approximate the gastric pouch. A gastrotomy is then performed on the posterior side of the gastric pouch and a jejunotomy is performed. Once this is done a gastrojejunal anastomosis is performed using a single fire of the linear stapler at 35 mm (Fig. 2). Once this is done a 34 French Gastric Lavage tube is advanced through the gastric pouch into the jejunum stenting the anastomosis.The common enterotomy is then closed in two layers over this tube with a 2-0 Vicryl. Once this is accomplished the bowel is divided as it enters the gastrojejunal anastomosis creating a biliary limb and an alimentary limb. About 100 cm distal on the alimentary limb the biliary limb is plugged back in to create a Roux-en-Y configuration. This is done in a side-to-side fashion after jejunotomies are performed utilizing a single fire of the linear stapler with a white load. The common enterotomy is closed with another fire of the stapler with a blue load; alternatively the common enterotomy can be closed with a 2-0 Vicryl. The mesenteric defect is closed using a 2-0 silk suture (Fig. 3). Petersen's space is closed using a 2-0 silk suture (Fig. 4). The gastrojejunal anastomosis is checked with an endoscope for hemostasis and an air leak test. This completes the procedure. Patient positioning and trocar position is illustrated in Figures 5 and 6.

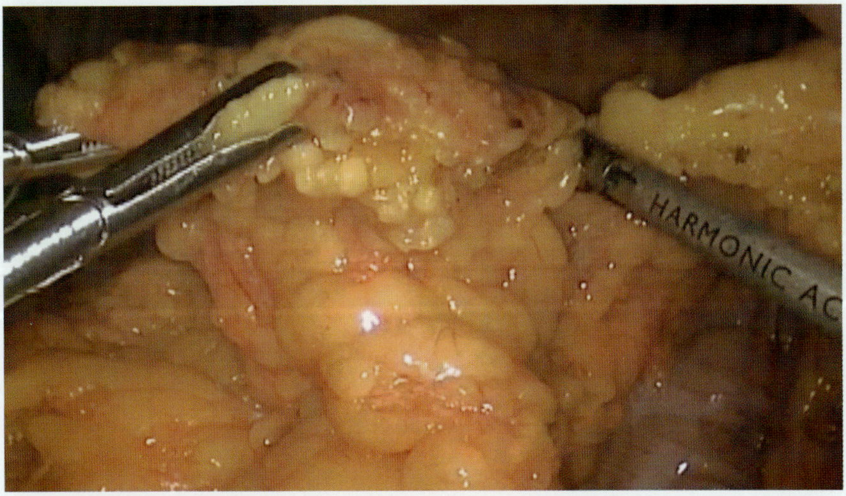

Fig. 1: Splitting greater omentum to allow passage of Roux limb.

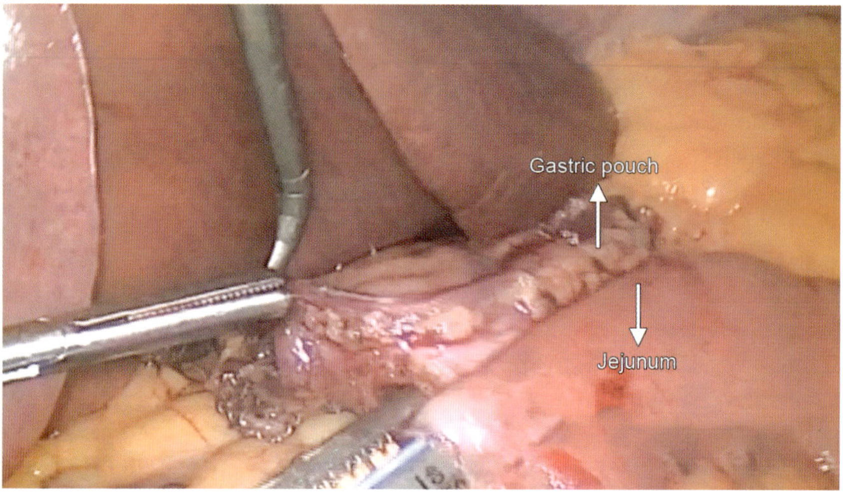

Fig. 2: Creation of gastrojejunal anastomosis using linear stapler.

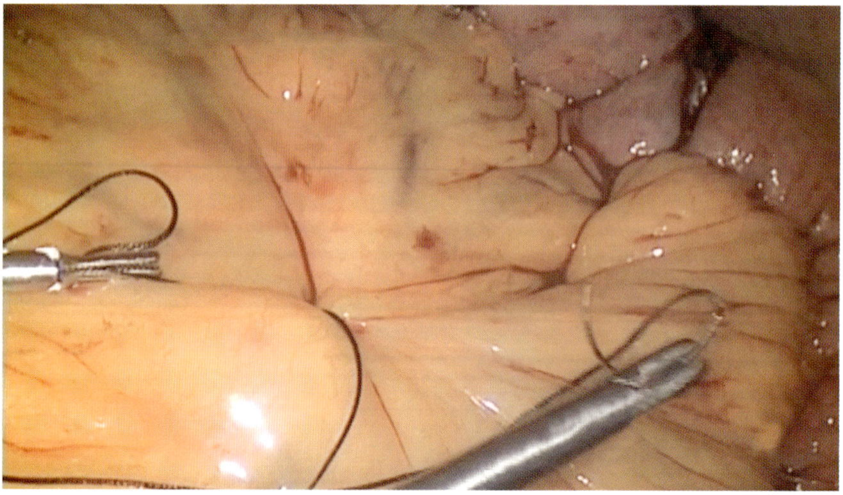

Fig. 3: Closure of jejunojejunal mesenteric defect.

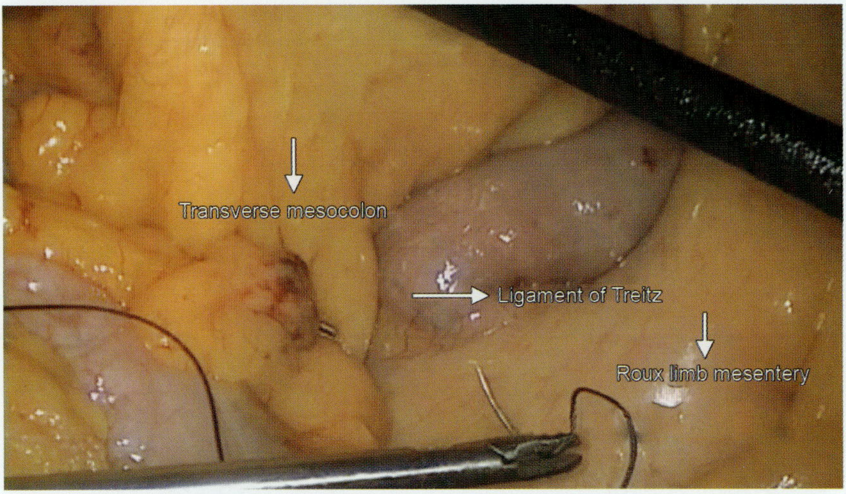

Fig. 4: Closure of Petersen's space.

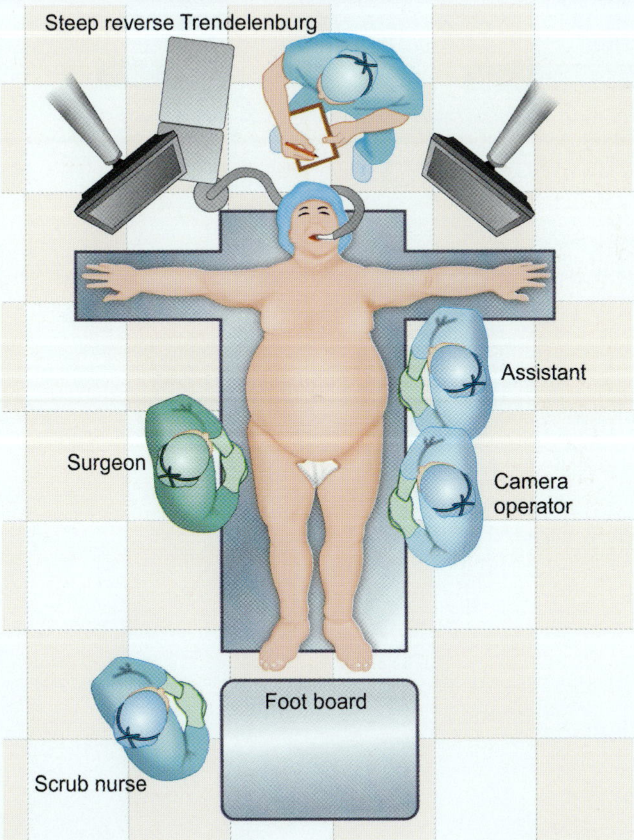

Fig. 5: Surgical positioning of patient.

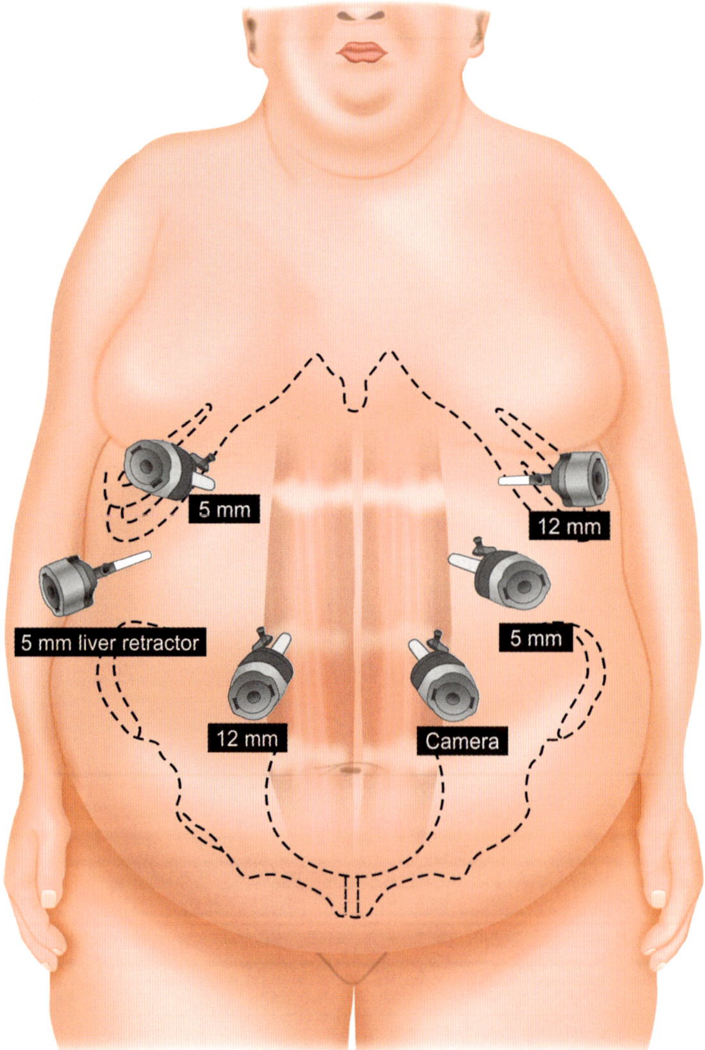

Fig. 6: Trocar position.

4 Laparoscopic Retrocolic Retrogastric Roux-en-Y Gastric Bypass

Rana C Pullatt, T Karl Byrne

OPERATIVE PROCEDURE

The patient is positioned supine with both arms out. An incision is made one open hand span width from the xiphoid process and two fingerbreadths to the left off the midline. This incision is deepened and the fascia is grasped with an Adair clamp. Pneumoperitoneum is introduced through a Veress needle to a pressure of 15 mm Hg. A 12 mm trocar is introduced through this. Diagnostic laparoscopy is performed. Alternatively in extremely obese patients a visual entry is done using a 12 mm trocar in the left subcostal region at Palmer's point using a visiport. A 5 mm trocar is placed just below the right costal margin in the anterior axillary line to introduce the liver retractor; alternatively the liver retractor can be placed just below the xiphoid process. A 5 mm trocar is placed on the right side just below the right costal margin at the mid clavicular line. A 12 mm trocar is placed one hand width below that slightly to the right side of the 5 mm trocar. Two other trocars are placed in the left side. One 12 mm trocar is placed in the left subcostal margin in the mid clavicular line. Another 5 mm trocar is placed one hand width below the 12 mm trocar. The angle of His is visualized and dissected. The left gastric artery is visualized. A small gastric pouch is created by transecting the stomach at the level of the second gastric vessel about 5 cm from the GE junction. The mesentery of the stomach is taken with the stapler. A green load is used for thick male stomachs and a blue load is usually used for female stomachs. The first fire of the stapler is done with staple line reinforcement. A small L shaped pouch is thus created based on the lesser curvature. Once complete division of the stomach is accomplished the posterior side of the gastric pouch is cleared off the fat and mesentery for an appropriate area for anastomosis. A penrose drain is attached to the gastric pouch to serve as a guide to bring the Roux limb in a retrocolic retrogastric fashion (Fig. 1). A window is made in the greater omentum and a retrogastric tunnel is made (Fig. 2). The ligament of Treitz is identified and the bowel is followed for

25 cm. The jejunum is transected with a single fire of the linear stapler with a white load. The mesentery is divided with an energy device. The alimentary limb is then advanced 100 cm, the biliary limb is then reanastomosed to the alimentary limb at this point in a Roux-en-Y configuration. This is done in a side-to-side fashion after jejunotomies are performed utilizing a single fire of the linear stapler with a white load. The common enterotomy is closed with another fire of the stapler with a blue load; alternatively the common enterotomy can be closed with a 2-0 Vicryl. The mesenteric defect is closed using a 2-0 silk suture. Just above and left of the ligament of Treitz the mesocolon is opened and the previously placed penrose drain in the lesser sac is identified and brought into the inframesocolic space (Fig. 3). The Roux limb is attached to the penrose drain and the Roux limb is brought to the gastric pouch using the penrose drain for traction. Once this is done, stay sutures may be placed if the anastomosis is to be performed to the anterior aspect of the gastric pouch, alternatively the anastomosis may be performed to the posterior aspect of the gastric pouch. A gastrostomy is then performed on the posterior side of the gastric pouch and a jejunotomy is performed. Once this is done a gastrojejunal anastomosis is performed using a single fire of the linear stapler at 35 mm. Once this is done a 34 French Gastric Lavage tube is advanced through the gastric pouch into the jejunum stenting the anastomosis. The common enterotomy is then closed in two layers over this tube with a 2-0 Polysorb. Petersen's space is closed using a 2-0 surgidac suture (Fig. 4). The gastrojejunal anastomosis is checked with an endoscope for hemostasis and an air leak test, this completes the procedure. Patient positioning and trocar position is illustrated in Figures 5 and 6.

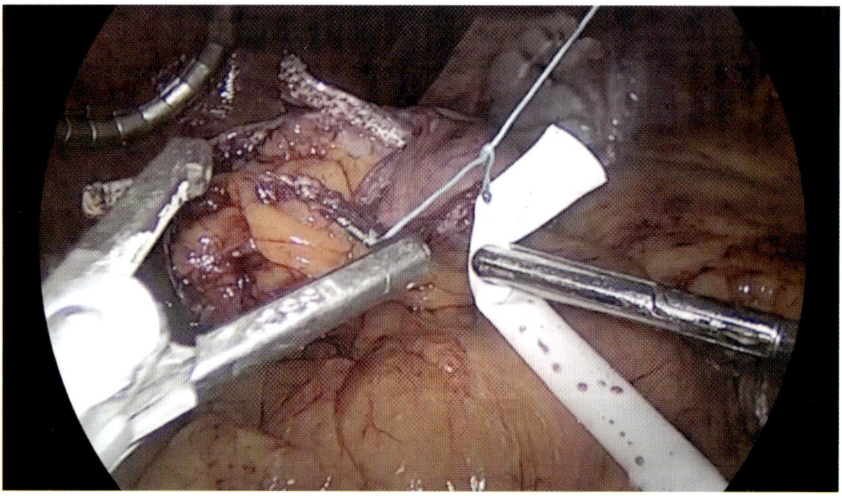

Fig. 1: Suturing penrose drain to gastric pouch.

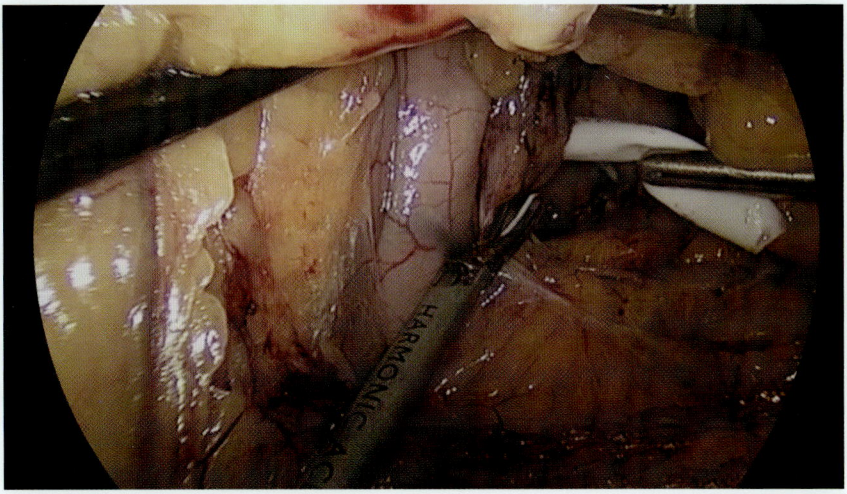

Fig. 2: Creation of retrogastric tunnel.

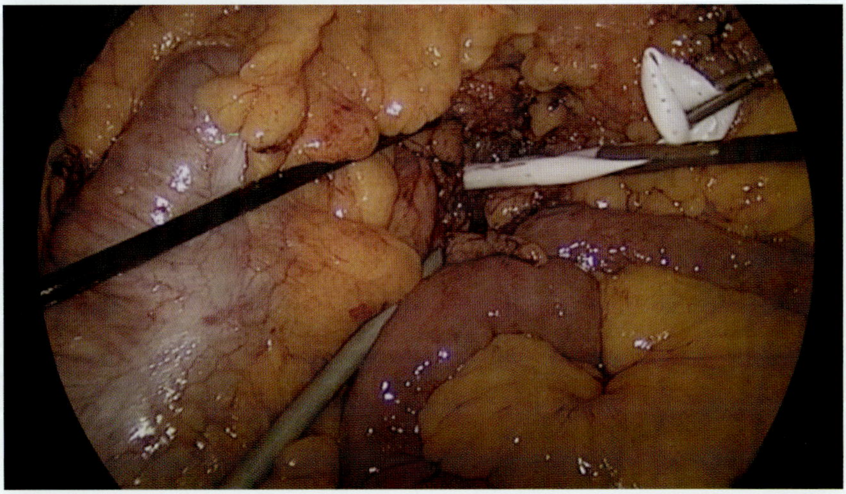

Fig. 3: Creation of mesocolic window.

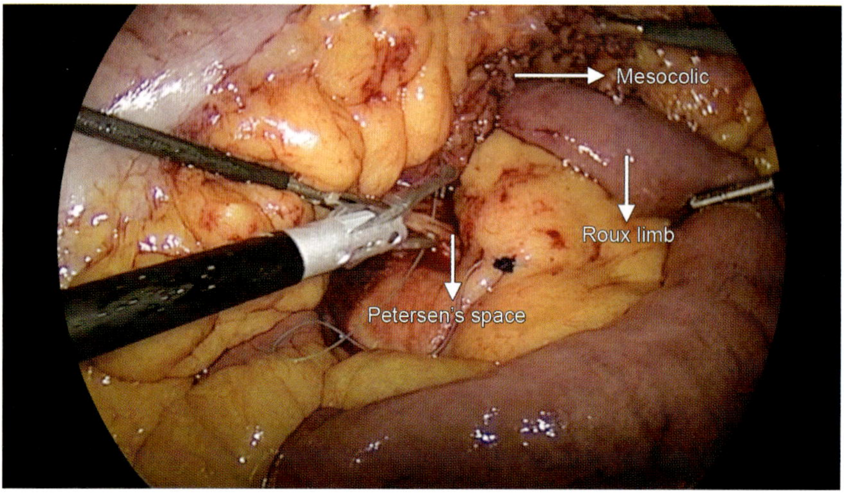

Fig. 4: Closure of Petersen's space.

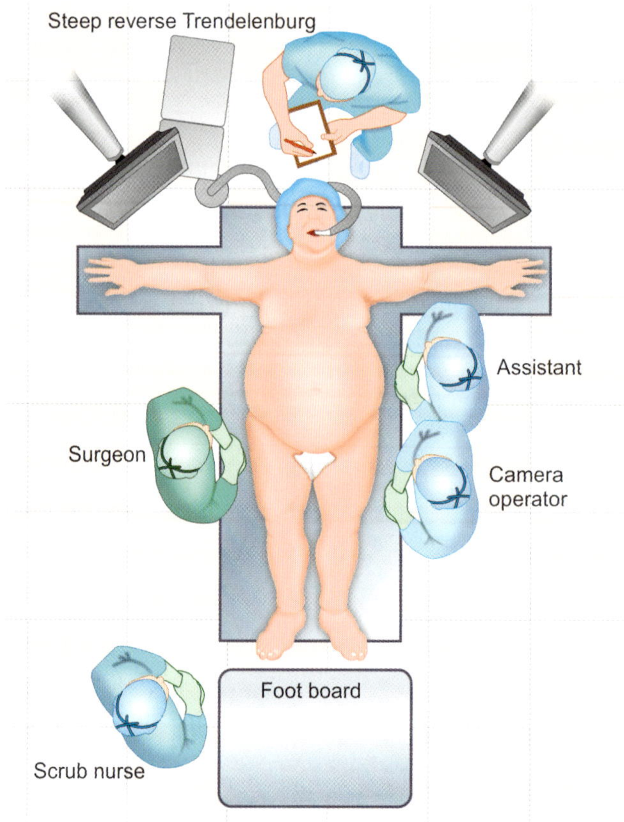

Fig. 5: Surgical positioning of patient.

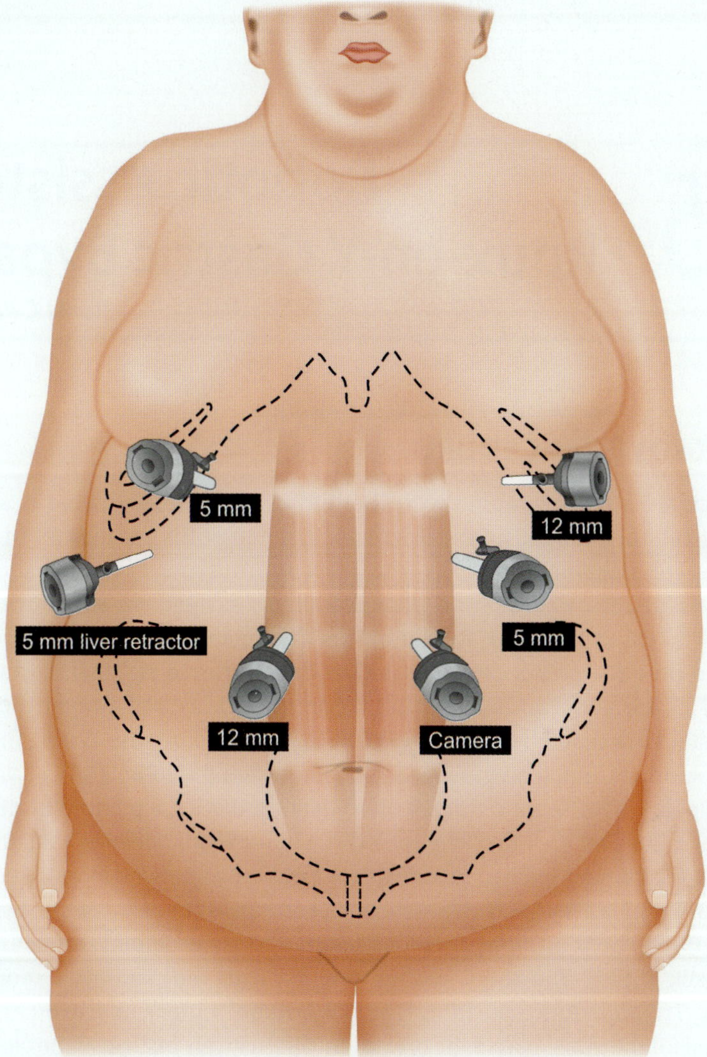

Fig. 6: Trocar position.

5 Robotic Assisted Roux-en-Y Gastric Bypass

Rana C Pullatt

OPERATIVE PROCEDURE

The patient is placed supine with the left arm tucked. The table is angled 20 degrees to the right from horizontal. The patient is positioned in steep reverse Trendelenburg position. The robot is brought over the left shoulder for docking. The camera port is placed after veress needle is introduced into the fascia just to the left of the umbilicus one open hands breath below the xiphoid process. A liver retractor is introduced from a right subcostal port placed in the anterior axillary line. A robotic trocar is placed in the right subcostal region in the mid clavicular line just below the costal margin. A 12 mm trocar is placed in the right side between the robotic trocar and the camera port. Two robotic trocars are placed in the left side, one in the mid clavicular line and the other one is placed a hand width lateral to that. Initially the robotic camera is introduced without the robot being docked. The ligament of Treitz is identified, a loop of bowel about 50 cm distal to the ligament is identified and is brought up and is secured to the excluded stomach using a 2-0 silk suture. The robot is then docked with the patient in moderate reverse Trendelenburg position (Fig. 1). A hook cautery and two cardieres are used for the initial part of the operation, alternatively instead of the cardieres double fenestrated graspers may be used. The angle of His is dissected and the lesser sac is opened. A small gastric pouch is created by division of the stomach below the left gastric vessels (Fig. 2). Generally three fires of the stapler are done to create a small gastric pouch, one horizontal and two vertical fires. The bowel loop which was previously secured to the excluded stomach is then released and a two layer anastomosis is performed with 2-0 vicryl sutures (Fig. 3). This is performed over a 34 Fr Ewald tube. The loop gastrojejunostomy is thus complete (Fig. 4). Once this is completed the loop of bowel is divided as it enters the gastric pouch creating a Roux limb and a biliary limb (Fig. 5). About 100 cm distal on the alimentary limb the biliary limb is plugged back in to create a Roux-en-Y configuration. This is done in a side-to-side fashion after jejunostomies are performed and a single fire of the linear stapler with a white load (Fig. 6). The common enterotomy is closed with another fire of the stapler with a blue load (Fig. 7); alternatively the common enterotomy can be closed with a 2-0 Vicryl. The mesenteric defect is closed using a 2-0 silk suture. Petersen's space is closed using a 2-0 silk suture. The gastrojejunal anastomosis is checked with an endoscope for hemostasis and an air leak test, this completes the procedure. Figures 8 and 9 demonstrate the schematic for the port positions and robot docking postion.

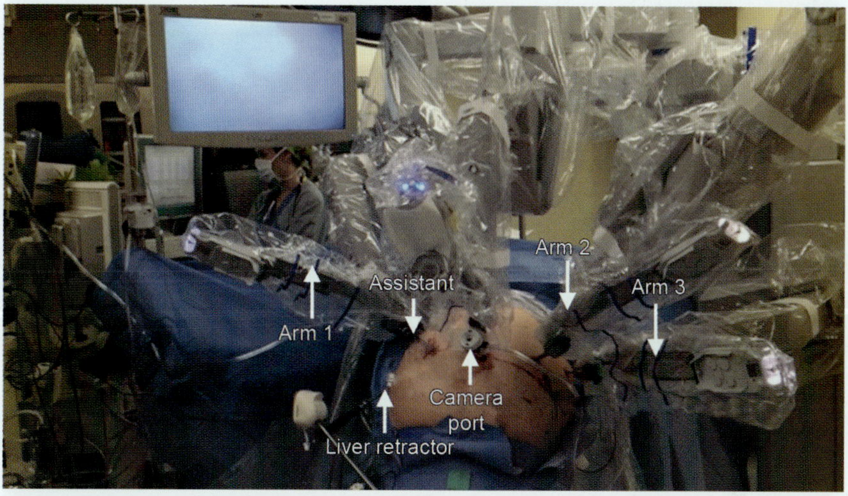

Fig. 1: Patient positon after docking the robot.

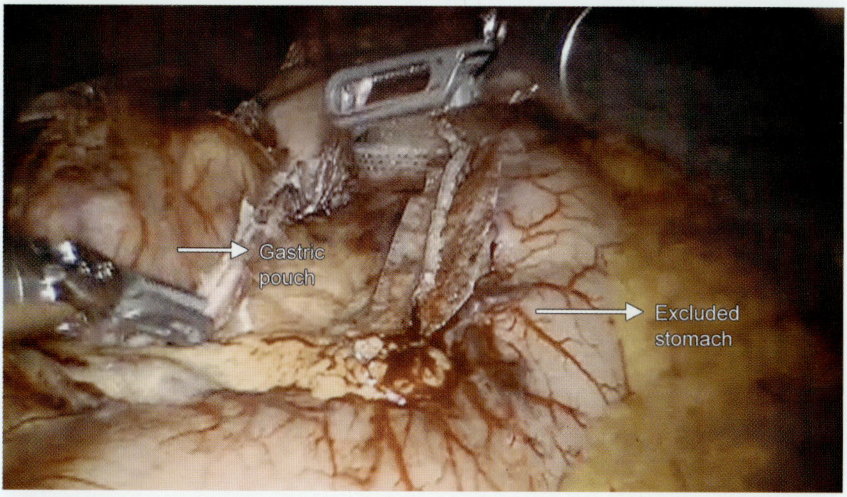

Fig. 2: Creation of gastric pouch.

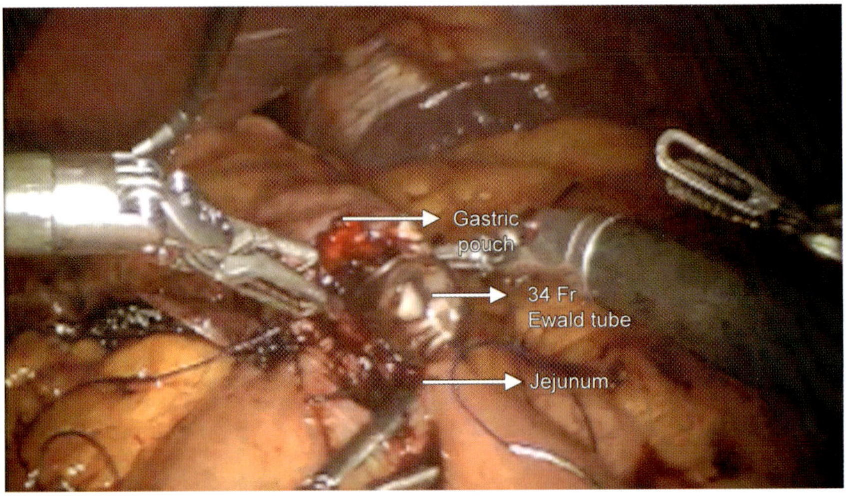

Fig. 3: Creation of gastrojejunostomy over 34 Fr Ewald tube.

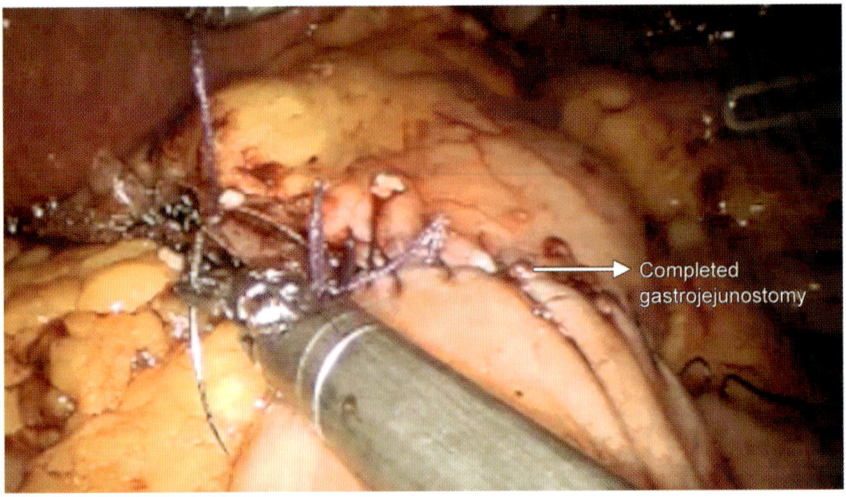

Fig. 4: Completed gastrojejunostomy.

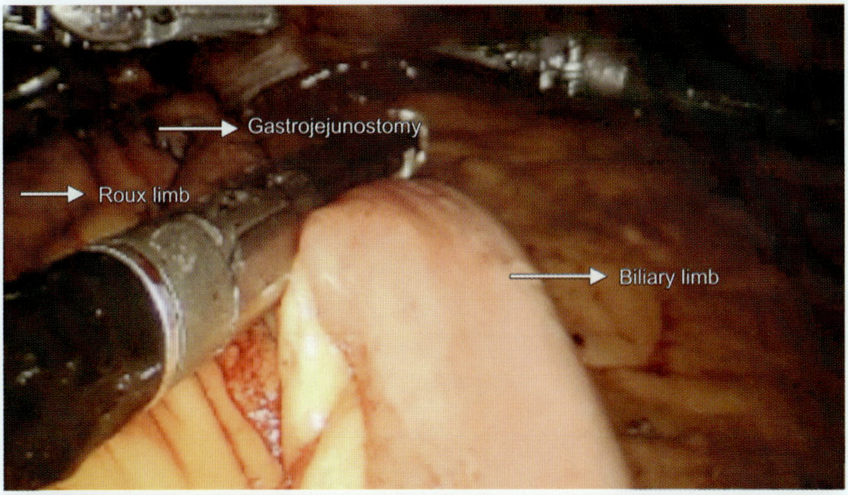

Fig. 5: Conversion of loop GJ to Roux configuration.

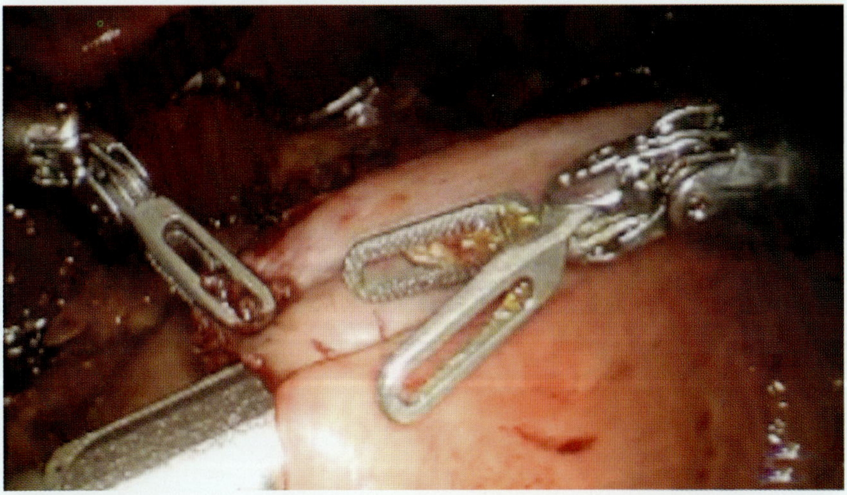

Fig. 6: Creation of jejunojejunostomy.

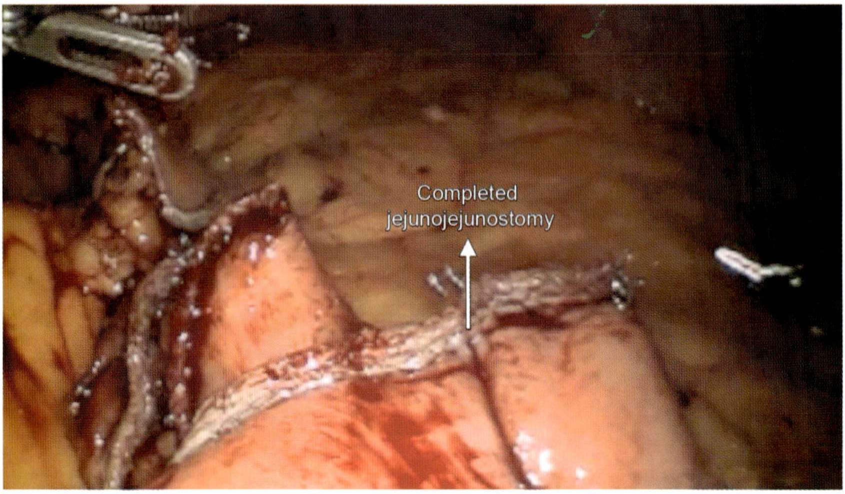

Fig. 7: Completed Jejunojejunostomy.

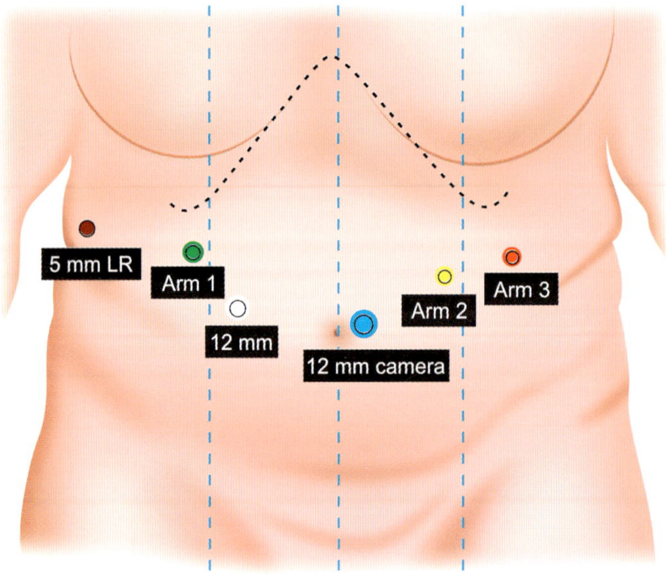

Fig. 8: Robotic gastric bypass trocar, camera and assistant port position.

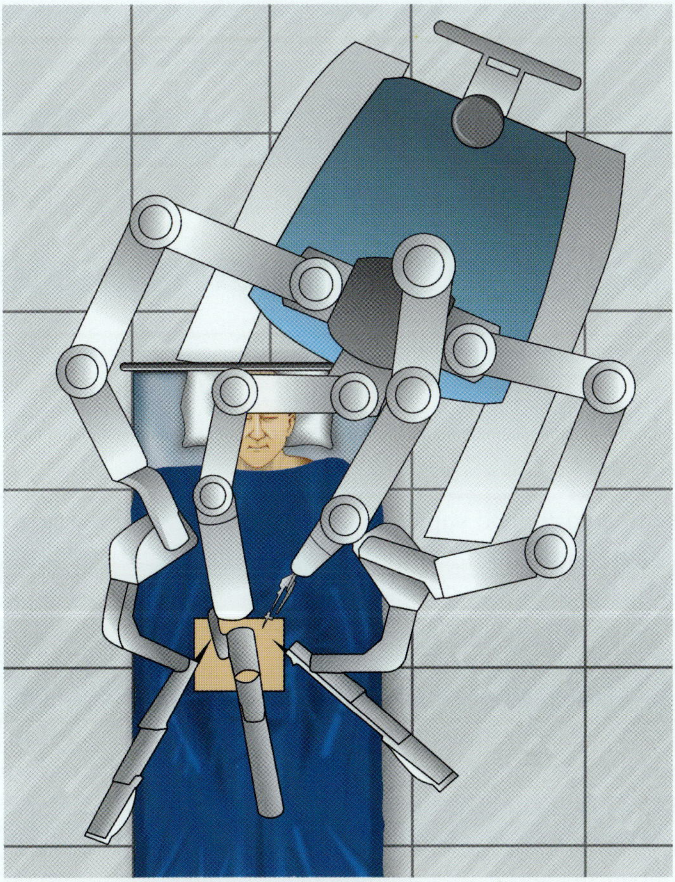

Fig. 9: Schematic representation of Robot docking in a 3-arm setup.

6 Laparoscopic Gastric Bypass—Circular Anastomosis Transgastric Method

John Scott

OPERATIVE PROCEDURE

The patient is positioned supine with both arms out. An incision is made 17 cm from the xiphoid process and 7 cm to the left off the midline. This incision is deepened, the fascia is grasped with an Adair clamp. Pneumoperitoneum is introduced through a Veress needle to a pressure of 15 mm Hg. A 12 mm trocar is introduced through this. Diagnostic laparoscopy is performed. A 5 mm trocar is placed just below the xiphoid to place a Nathanson Liver retractor. A 12 mm trocar is placed on the right side just below the right costal margin lateral to the mid clavicular line. Another 12 mm trocar is placed just to the right of the midline at the level of the camera trocar. Two other 12 mm trocars are placed on the left side (Fig. 5).

The Anvil of the 25 EEA is introduced through a gastrotomy on the stomach and the spike on the Anvil is used as a guide to make a counter incision on the upper stomach in the location of the future gastric pouch to position the Anvil in the appropriate place (Fig. 1). The angle of His is visualized and dissected. A small gastric pouch is created by transecting the stomach at the level of the second gastric vessel about 5 cm from the GE junction in a perigastric fashion below the Anvil. A small L shaped pouch is thus created based on the lesser curvature (Fig. 2). The small bowel is transected at 50 cm from the ligament of Treitz to create a Roux limb. The end of the Roux limb is then opened. The EEA stapler is then introduced after the 12 mm trocar in the left subcostal region is removed and brought in through the Roux limb and the spike is deployed and the stapler is mated creating the GJ anastomosis (Fig. 3). The anastomosis is inspected for hemostasis and the dog-ear of the Roux limb is transected flush to the GJ completing the anastomosis (Fig. 4). The anastomosis is reinforced with interrupted 2-0 PDS sutures and then tested with methylene blue. The remainder of the operation is completed in standard fashion.

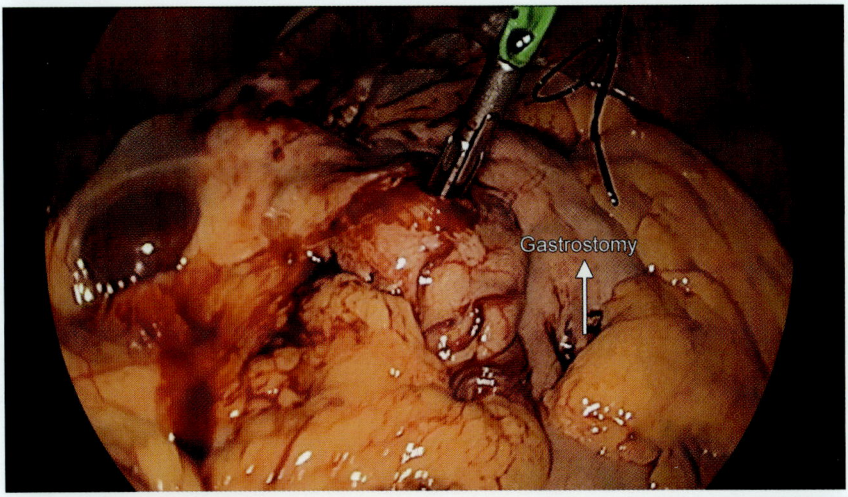

Fig. 1: Transgastric introduction of EEA Anvil.

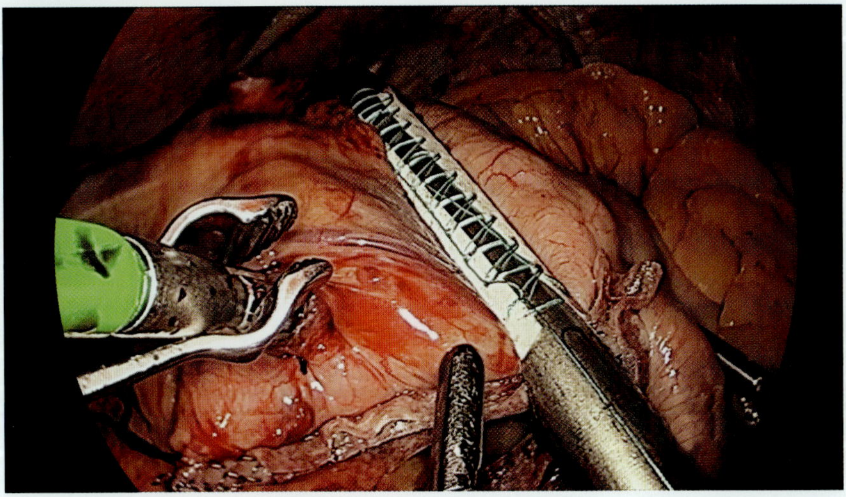

Fig. 2: Creation of gastric pouch.

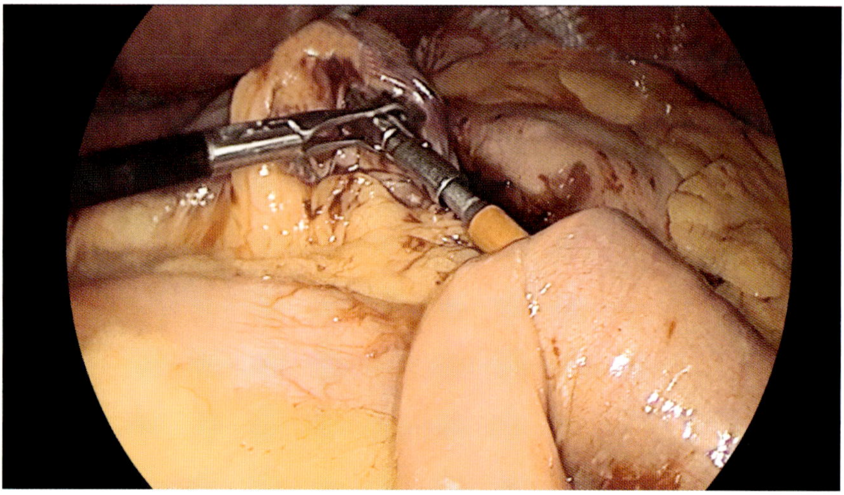

Fig. 3: Mating of EEA 25 stapler to create gastrojejunostomy.

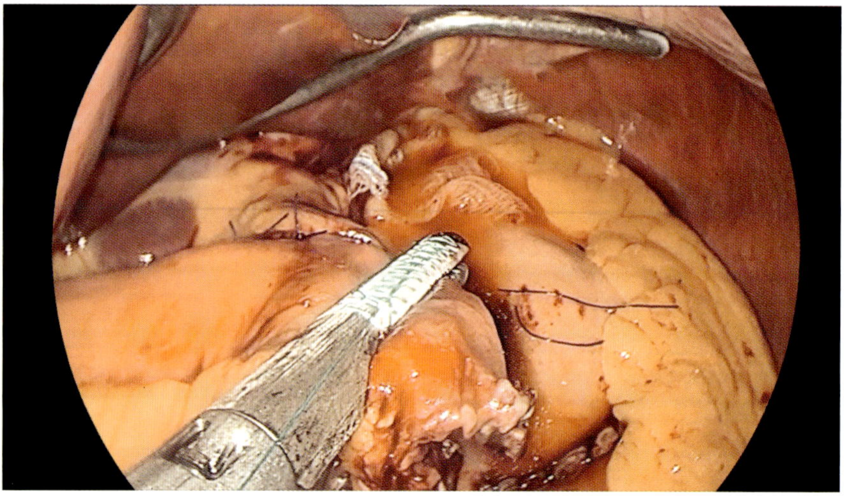

Fig. 4: Excision of dog-ear of Roux limb.

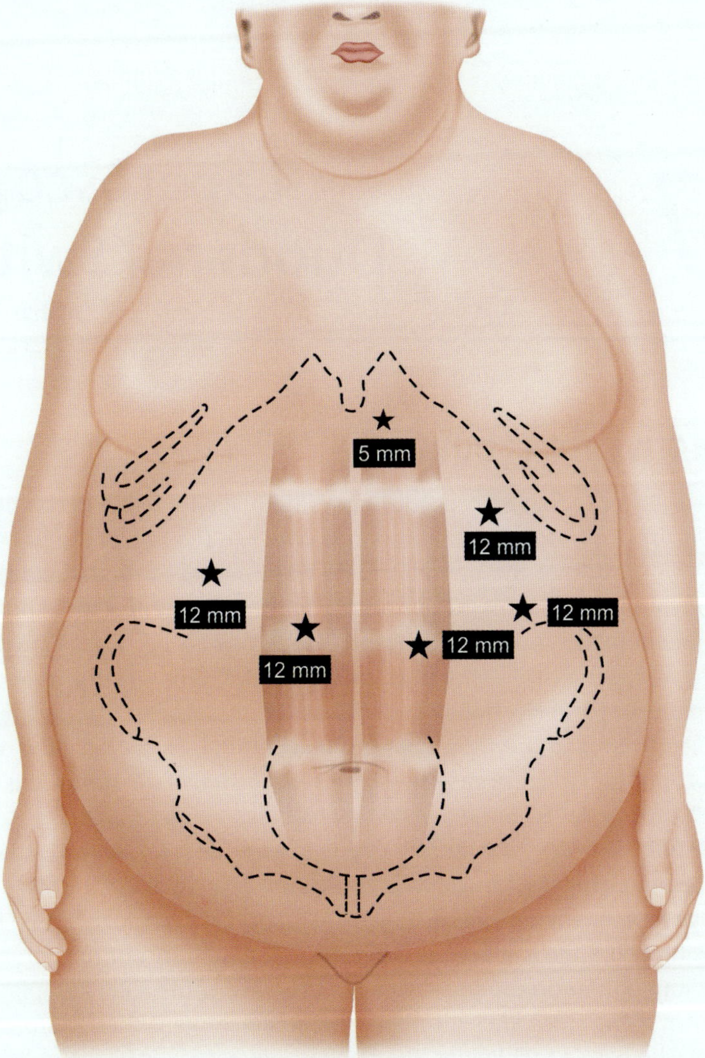

Fig. 5: Port position.

7 Laparoscopic Duodenal Switch

Mitch Roslin

OPERATIVE PROCEDURE

Six ports are used for the procedure and are placed as seen in the illustration (Fig. 4). The surgeon initially stands between the legs of the patient for the Sleeve portion of the operation and then moves to the left side of the position for the creation of the common channel. The surgeon then performs the duodenoileostomy from between the legs. The procedure begins by creating a sleeve gastrectomy in standard fashion (Fig. 1). The lesser sac is entered; the angle of His is dissected till the left crus is seen. The pars flaccida is opened to look at the right crus to make sure no hiatal hernia is visualized. As opposed to sleeve gastrectomy the dissection of the stomach is continued till the pylorus is elevated. A 40 French bougie is placed into the stomach and advanced to the antrum hugging the lesser sac. A sleeve gastrectomy is performed using the bougie as a guide. The first fire is done with a black cartridge followed by a green cartridge and then a gold cartridge is used for the upper stomach. Care is taken, as in a sleeve gastrectomy not to encroach on the GE junction or on the incisura angularis. The entire sleeve staple line is over sown using a 2-0 PDS suture. A cholecystectomy is then performed in patients who have a gallbladder. The duodenal dissection is begun on the right side of where the common duct passes superiorly (Fig. 2). This will eventually serve as the target for where the stapler will exit during duodenal transection. Pyloric dissection is continued inferiorly till a plane is developed beneath the duodenum. The duodenum is then transected using a blue load stapler creating a 3–4 cm duodenal cuff. The omentum is then divided to create a pathway for the Roux limb. The surgeon then moves to the left of the patient. The terminal ileum is located; 125 cm of the small bowel is measured from the terminal ileum. The bowel is rotated in an anticlockwise direction and at the 125 cm mark on the antimesenteric border an enterotomy is made. Another 175 cm of the bowel is then counted upstream by rotating the bowel in anticlockwise direction and rotating it superiorly to the patient's right to keep the proper orientation. The bowel is then divided with a white load at this point approximately 300 cm for the ileocecal junction. The left hand of the surgeon is positioned on the proximal biliopancreatic end and the right hand is positioned on the eventual Roux limb. An enterotomy is then performed about 6 cm from the end of the biliopancreatic limb to allow for enough space for eventual firing of the stapler both proximally and distally to create a H shaped anastomosis for the eventual enteroenterostomy. The Roux limb is then rotated in an anti-clockwise direction in close proximity to the biliopancreatic limb. This will eventually line up the enterotomy on the biliopancreatic limb to the initial enterotomy created on the bowel 75 cm from the ileocecal junction. Once these are lined up the anastomosis is created in a H shaped fashion by firing the stapler proximally and distally and the common enterotomy is closed perpendicular to the initial staple line to prevent narrowing of the anastomosis. The surgeon then moves back between the legs of the patient and the Roux limb is brought up in the correct orientation without twisting. The end of the Roux limb and its mesentery face medially. A 2 cm duodenotmy and an enterotomy are made after stay sutures are placed in the ends. The anastomosis is done in 2 layers using 2-0 PDS suture. The anastomosis is completed using methylene blue and the procedure is thus complete (Fig. 3).

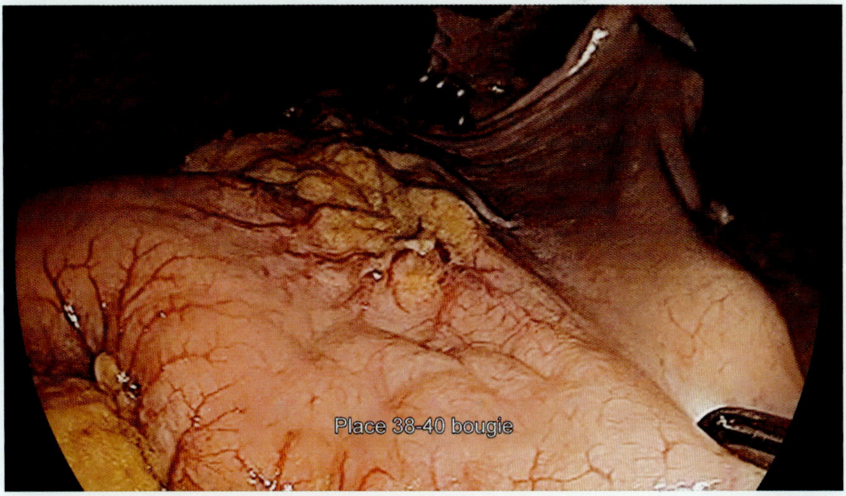

Fig. 1: Creation of sleeve gastrectomy.

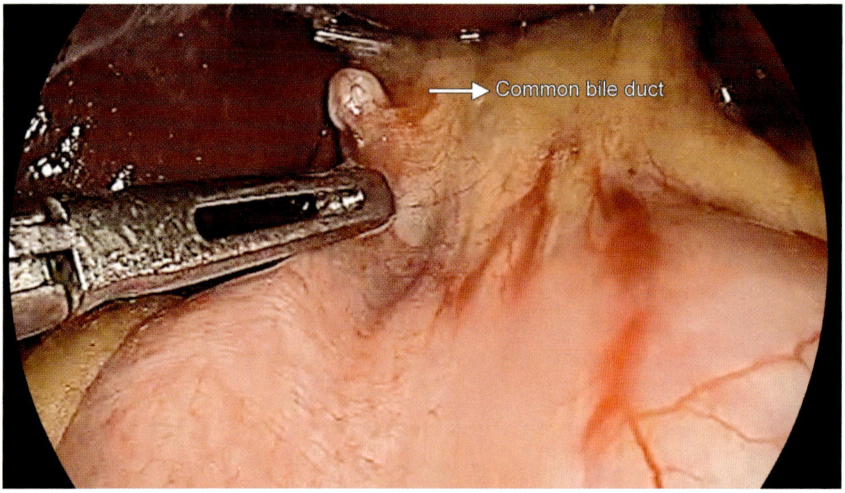

Fig. 2: Postpyloric dissection.

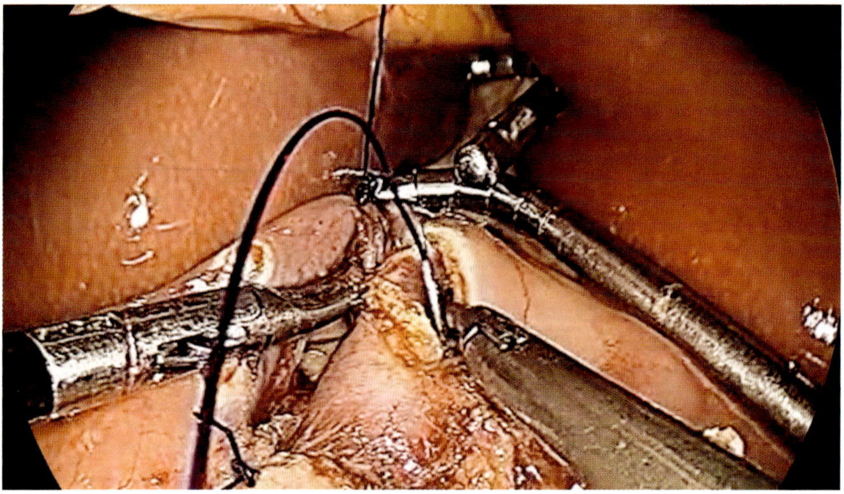

Fig. 3: Duodenoileal anastomosis.

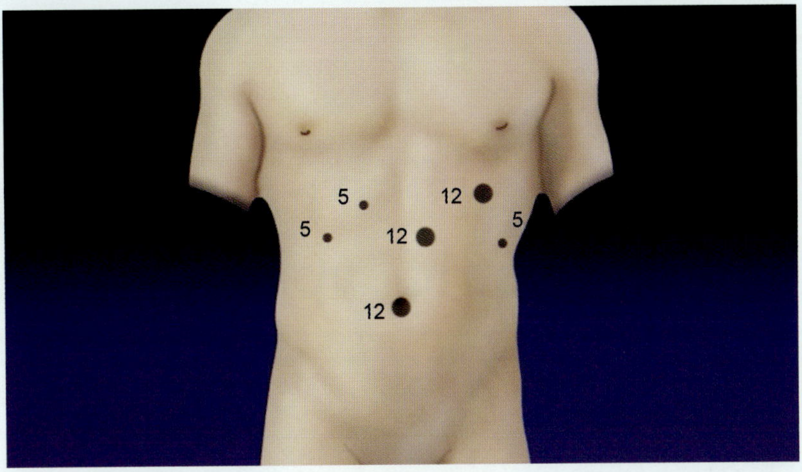

Fig. 4: Port position.

8 ERCP in Roux-en-Y Gastric Bypass Patients

Rana C Pullatt, Greg Cote

OPERATIVE PROCEDURE

A 12 mm or 5 mm camera trocar is placed in standard fashion just to the left of midline. Two 5 mm trocars are placed in the right side. Another 5 mm trocar is placed in the left side. A gastrotomy is performed in the excluded stomach and the 12 mm balloon trocar or a 15 mm trocar is introduced through the gastrotomy. If a 12 mm balloon trocar is used then no fixation to the stomach is required (Fig. 1). The 12 mm trocars only accommodate the older ERCP scopes. However, if a standard ERCP scope is used then a 15 mm trocar is required to accommodate the scope. The 15 mm trocar does not come with a self-retaining balloon configuration at this time and so the trocar is fixed to the stomach with a purse string suture with a 2-0 Vicryl. The surgical field is then draped with a hole cut out in the drape to accommodate the 12 mm trocar in the excluded stomach and the ERCP is completed (Fig. 2). The gastrotomy is closed in two layers with a 2-0 Vicryl suture. This completes the procedure. Port positions are described in Figure 3.

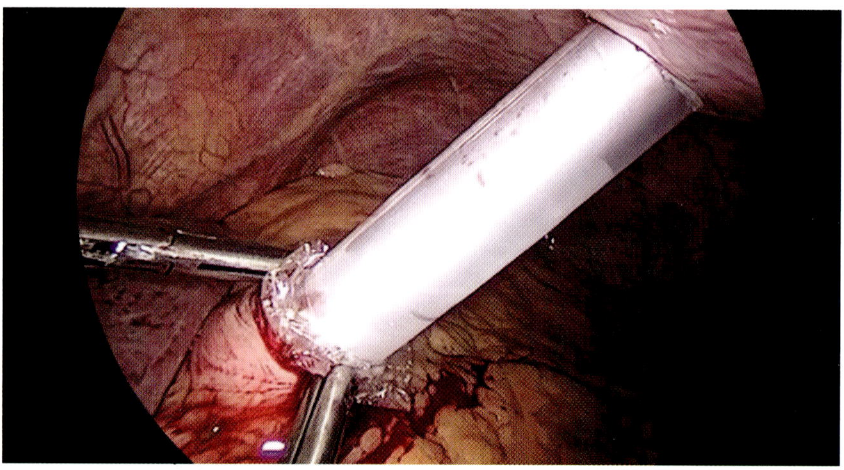

Fig. 1: Creation of gastrostomy in excluded stomach to introduce trocar.

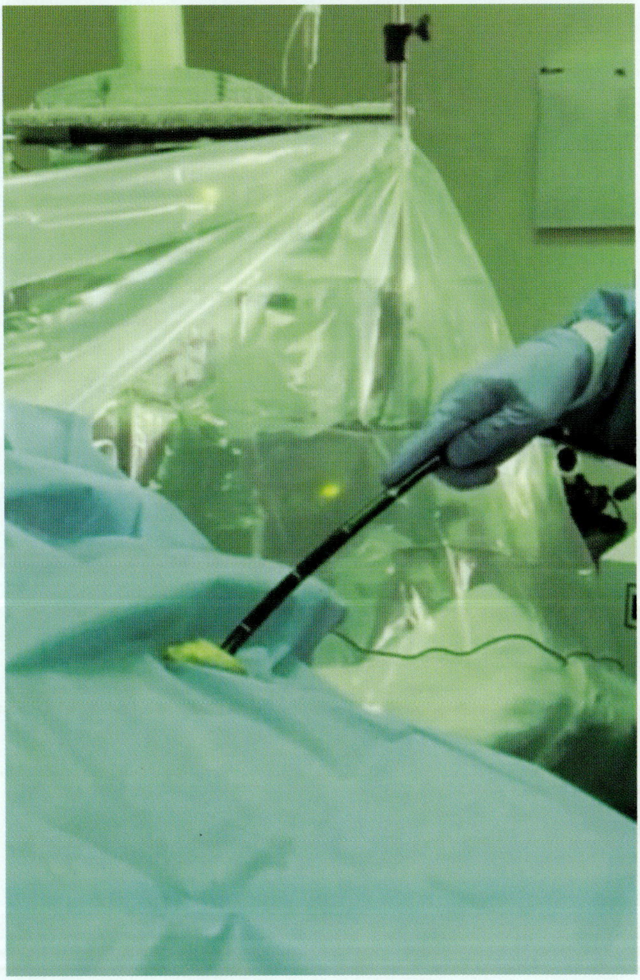

Fig. 2: Introduction of ERCP scope.

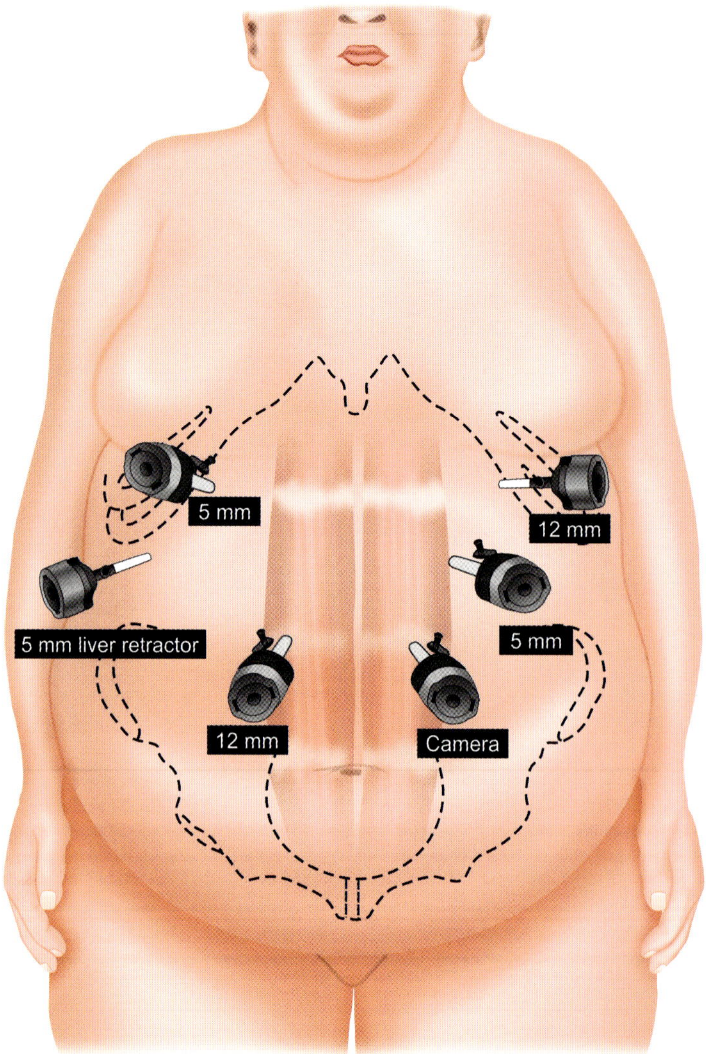

Fig. 3: Port positions.

9 SIPS (Stomach, Intestine and Pylorus Sparing Surgery)

Mitch Roslin

OPERATIVE PROCEDURE

Six ports are used for the procedure and are placed as seen in the illustration (Fig. 5). The surgeon initially stands between the legs of the patient for the sleeve portion of the operation and then moves to the left side of the position for measuring the bowel from the ileocecal junction. The surgeon then performs the duodenoileostomy from between the legs. The first step of the procedure is to create a sleeve gastrectomy over a 42 French bougie (Fig. 1). Once the sleeve is complete, the gastroepiploic vessels are taken down from the end of the sleeve staple line past the pylorus to where the perforating vessels from the pancreas enter the duodenum. This is almost always 2 to 3 cm beyond the pylorus. A blunt instrument is passed behind the duodenum to create a path for the division of the duodenum. The duodenum is now divided with a stapler (Fig. 2). If a cholecystectomy is planned, it is performed at this time.

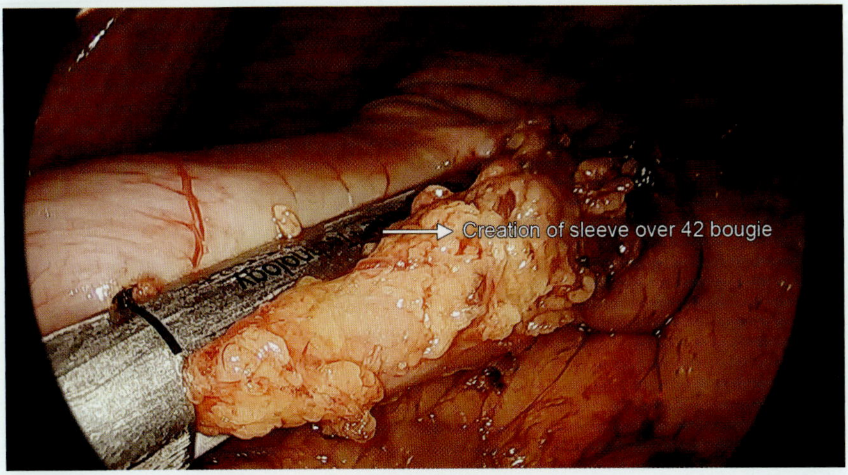

Fig. 1: Creation of sleeve.

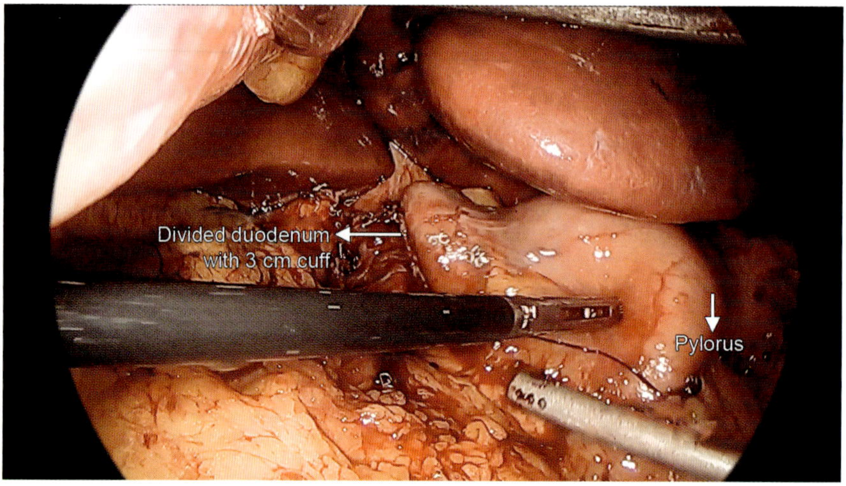

Fig. 2: Postpyloric duodenal division.

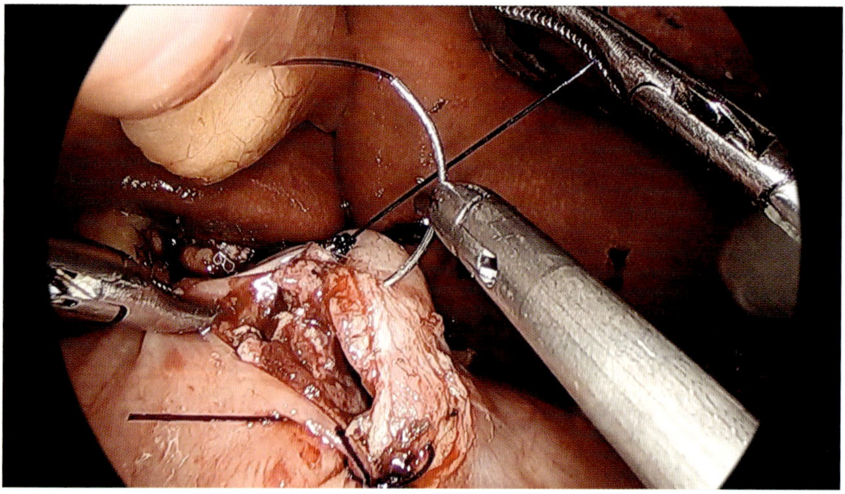

Fig. 3: Creation of duodenoileostomy.

The terminal ileum is now located, and 3 meters of small bowel are measured. The mesenteric border of the bowel at this point is attached to the end of the proximal duodenum staple line using an absorbable suture. The loop is set up so the efferent limb is descending on the patient's right, and the afferent limb is ascending coming up from the left. A duodenotomy and enterotomy are made that are approximately 2 cm. The enterotomy is as big as technically possible since it plays no role in the weight loss of the procedure. The enterotomy is closed with a running posterior layer and a running anterior layer (Fig. 3). The anastomosis is tested intraoperatively for leak (Fig. 4).

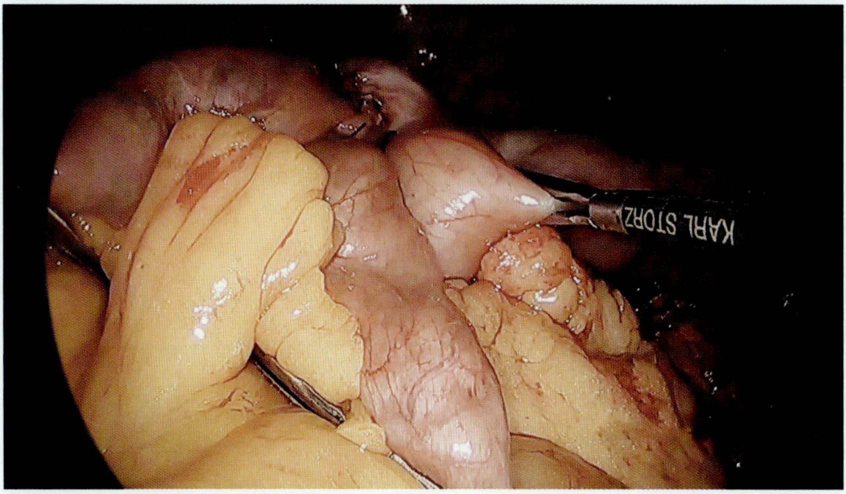

Fig. 4: Leak test with methylene blue.

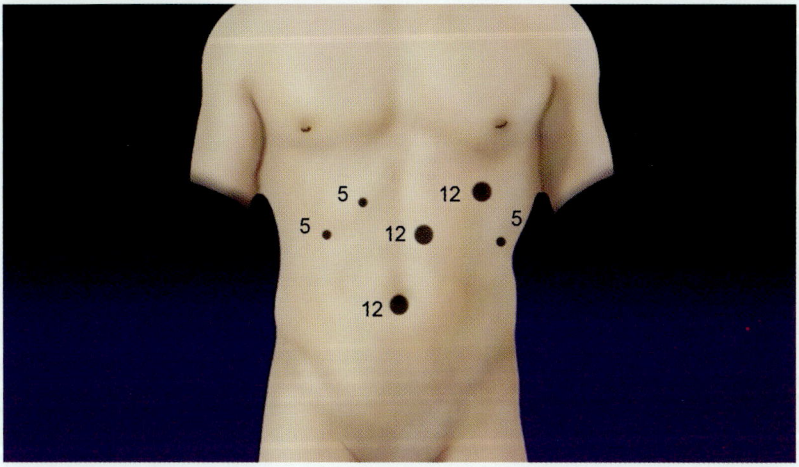

Fig. 5: Port positions.

Index

Note: Page numbers followed by *f* refer to figure.

S